TEACHER'S MANUAL

for

Building Construction and Design

TEACHER'S MANUAL

for

Building Construction and Design

James Ambrose
University of Southern California

VNR SPRINGER SCIENCE+BUSINESS MEDIA, LLC

16 15 14 13 12 11 10 9 8 7 6 5 4 3 2 1

Contents

Preface

This publication is intended for persons who are planning to use my book, **Building Construction and Design**, as a basic text or reference for some teaching effort. The book was indeed written to be used for study purposes, including those involving some classroom situation with a teacher. The book itself is organized and presented essentially for the utility of the readers; with or without the benefit of guidance by a teacher. This manual is written for the teacher and deals with teaching in general, as well as with the specific use of my book.

The preparation of the book - and of this manual - come forth after some 50 years of work by me in building construction; ranging from actual construction labor to professional design, teaching, and writing. The book is intended to share that experience with the generally uninformed but motivated reader, having a basic interest in the design of buildings. However, there are many ways to use the book for particular forms of study or teaching. This manual explores the various possibilities for using the book in just about all the ways I can imagine in terms of teaching situations and learning goals.

Most college teachers get no teacher education or training (me included). If both totally unprepared by training and also inexperienced in teaching work, the teacher faces a vast abyss of unknowns in approaching the classroom and the blank stares of a room full of students. Any help is wanted, and this manual may hopefully supply some for the less experienced teachers. In addition to a lot of discussion, there are many samples of typical course schedules, assignments, quizzes and exams; all related specifically to the use of my book. Surely the creative educator will quickly develop some original approaches, but meanwhile, here is some very time-tested, generic teaching material. Teach; learn; enjoy!

James Ambrose

1

Introduction

1.1 About Me

This manual is about how to use my book for various purposes in teaching building construction. While the book itself stands as the primary evidence of my involvement, it may behoove the reader to consider somewhat where I come from in terms of experience, attitudes, and involvements in the subject. To that end, I offer the following short bio.

My earliest involvement in construction started at age 12 when I got my first job as a construction worker (mason's helper). Never mind child labor laws, it was the Great Depression. I also pursued all the offerings available in school in drafting, which then included three years before, and four years during high school. All of that before entering architecture school.

Despite the school work, and for purely economic reasons, my money-earning work continued to be in construction jobs - from laborer to scab carpenter. Even during my service in the US Army, although they put my architectural training to work by having me design some buildings, it worked out that - where we were in Korea at the time - there were no people who could read my drawings. So, I had to also **build** the buildings. A traumatic experience indelibly etched in my memory.

Subsequently, I finally finished architecture school (architectural engineering, actually) and worked as a structural designer/draftsman, working up to project engineer in a large architecture office. Out of a combination of freak opportunity and job burnout, I took my first teaching position at my alma mater, the U. of Illinois at Urbana, in 1959. Thirty-three years later, I am still at it, trying to squeeze some things into the skulls of architecture students.

Along the way since graduating from the U. of Illinois, I have accumulated a variety of professional experiences and licenses in the fields of architecture and structural engineering. Although I have now given up professional practice (including the phone calls, lawsuits, etc.), I still have vivid memories of many encounters in the office, the field, and other places of battle.

In my first semester of teaching, I found it necessary to supplement the text I was assigned to use with some of my own class notes. In subsequent semesters the notes grew - eventually outweighing the text. At that point, I decided to write my own text(s), and my writing/publishing career was launched.

This book - **Building Construction and Design** - represents my first major departure from the subject area of my previous writing, which was essentially investigation and design of building structures. You understand - I have worked, studied, and professionally practiced in building construction since the age of 12! But my writing in the fully engaged topic started with this book. (Actually with its predecessors, which were the four-book series on the topic.)

So - that's where I come from. I have taught just about every topic except history in the architecture curriculum (including design studios) and have written some kind of text materials for most of the courses. With that behind me, I offer the advice in this manual for use by teachers who may consider using my book.

1.2   Why I Wrote the Book

I had a number of personal reasons for writing this book. What I mean to address here is what motivated me to write it in this particular form. This had to do somewhat with setting the book apart from other current texts, but also with some particular issues I had in mind for such a book.

First and foremost - as it says repeatedly in the book - it is developed from a **designer's** point of view. Building construction as a topic is enormous if all approaches and all subjects are addressed. This book assumes that an interest in building design precedes the need for concerns about the technology and methods of construction. Thus, the pursuit of information about construction essentially comes up within the basic process of building design.

With this primary concern, I felt it necessary to present a number of examples of situations that occur in ordinary design work. A process that repeatedly occurs is that where a building scheme (preliminary design) is developed in the form of plans, elevations, and views that define a building's form and appearance. This is sufficient to explain the visible building (inside and out) and its arrangement of spaces and items. Many building designs are essentially "sold" to design clients on the basis of such studies.

Once sold, of course, the designer (or somebody) must proceed to figure out how to build it and go on to develop the necessary instructions to the builders (complete construction drawings and specs). The nine case studies in Chapter Ten of the book pick up the story at the end of the preliminary sketches and proceed to a sort of definitive design of the typical elements of the construction. Some of the considerations in this development are discussed in the text in Chapter Ten, but they also draw on the individual topic presentations in the earlier chapters.

The building construction shell (walls, roof, floors) cannot be developed without major considerations for the full incorporation of the various building subsystems (structure, HVAC, lighting, etc.). In this regard, some presentation is made in my book of the schemes and some significant details of the various subsystems; especially those that often have some notable impact on decisions about the building form and the general construction.

For my own teaching purposes, Chapter Ten is the key chapter, and I use the preceding materials as background for the most part. The extent of need for that "background" depends largely on the students being taught. Beginners need a lot of basic preparation; advanced students maybe very little.

So that is how the book is intended to work: as a vehicle for involving students in a process of figuring out the construction for a building. The example building may be one of the cases in my Chapter Ten, one of a similar type with the same basic considerations of use and scale, or a whole different example - such as one designed for a studio assignment. The student is thus first engaged in a study of a familiar form - a whole building as defined by use and shape. We then dissect the corpse to analyze its parts and proceed to reassemble it in detail.

I think this whole view is important, and to my knowledge is not much presented elsewhere in the literature. While the materials in Chapter Ten do not consist of actual complete construction drawings and specs, they do present a reasonably complete view of the building in whole and in part for a comprehensive grasp of the basic construction.

The first nine chapters of the book contain treatments of various aspects of the subject of building construction. Most fundamental issues are raised and a full treatment would produce a reasonable basic background in the subject. I think the basic ingredients are there for a whole development of the subject - at least as far as architects and other designers of buildings are concerned.

Study of particular single topics can be pursued through outside readings, field trips, class discussions, or supplementary teaching aids (slides, movies, samples, etc.). Later chapters in this manual give examples of courses that can be developed for these purposes.

For all its size, however, this book is a very brief sample of the whole topic of building construction. For some viability, it assumes that the teacher and students have access to some very standard references, such as **Sweets Catalog Files** and **Architectural Graphic Standards**, as well as various other current texts on construction. In other words, common references that you would expect to be in an architecture school library or somewhere in any large design office. My book does not remotely attempt, therefore, to be a self-contained source of endless detail about the subject of building materials and processes.

As a matter of fact, I consider it vital to get the students used to the idea that **they** have to go out and find information that is not provided in the text or classroom in order to complete assignments. Learning to find that information may be the single most useful accomplishment from the course efforts. Feeding them everything they need really defeats that purpose. Of course, you need to be sure that they can actually find some necessary information or it is not a fair game.

Well, that is what I had in mind for the book. At this moment of writing, I have not tried the book out myself, so I don't really know how successful it is. I expect, however, based on my umpteen years of experience, that I will end up using some supplementary materials to help out for the course, even though it is my own book. Architects are congenitally resistant to being fully contained with regard to their futures as designers in some established package. A wrapped-up deal is always a challenge; eliciting endless retries and criticisms. I expect to really butcher this book up in the second edition; based on my own experiences, if not on other's.

1.3 Why I Wrote the Teaching Manual

Every teacher who writes textbooks tends to model them to some extent around their own teaching experiences and involvements. It is hard to develop a text that lends itself to many courses; of different form, duration, and specific orientation. Still, a text that presents a generally developed subject in a fundamental way can usually be used to some degree for many different purposes.

Besides presenting some of my own observations and experiences in 33 years of teaching, this manual is intended to show how my book can be used for some very common courses (in architecture programs), but also for a variety of teaching purposes. Face it, I want to sell the book to a wide market.

More practically, I want to provide teachers with some sample course materials to make it easier to make up a course around my book. Many teachers have little experience, and typically little guidance, in the organization of a course. I want to help them do the dirty work: making a class schedule, writing a course syllabus, writing assignments, quizzes, and exams. I can't help with the worst part - the grading - but I hope what is here may be useful.

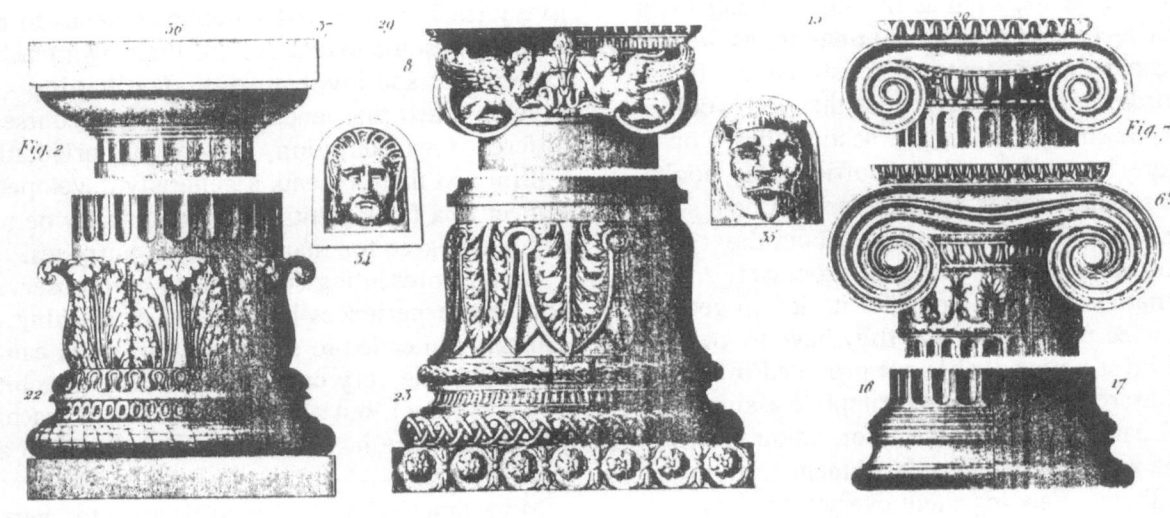

2

Teaching and Learning

If you will pardon me, I will make an assumption here: that the vast majority of you who are bothering to read this manual have probably never had five minutes of useful instruction about how to teach. Me either. I won't break your record much here, but will try to address some very basic considerations about the general task of teaching and about the more critical concern - learning.

2.1 Teaching Tasks and Responsibilities

You can't really **make** people learn. But you can try to inspire, cajole, persuade, or - when all else fails - threaten them into studying. On various occasions I try all of these approaches; but always use fear when it is available to me. For students in a credit-earning course I always keep the specter of flunking readily at hand.

The fundamental responsibilities of a teacher are the following:

1. To clearly define a body of subject material and the goals for the course of study; in other words, what the course is going to try to accomplish.

2. To clearly indicate what it is that you expect the students to do and when.

3. To assure that the students have the necessary resources to accomplish what you are asking of them; through some combination of classroom lectures and discussions, texts and handouts, available references, etc.

4. To provide them as best you can with the necessary advice and counselling they need while pursuing the work.

5. And then to be as tough as you can in dumping on them when they don't do the work right and/or on time.

If you know the subject at least a little more than the students and have any reasonable ability to organize, you can accomplish the first three of these with some effort. Item four is often a challenge, frustrated by students who do not come to class, by students who are too shy to ask questions, and by simple logistics if you have a large class.

Item five is fraught with difficulty, principally by the following:

Your own will, resolve, and thin skin.

The student's ability to cheat and weasel.

Give students any excuse: the war, the weather, gender, cultural heritage, health, religion, studio

5

charrettes - and they will extrapolate it into a catastrophe of endless proportions, justifying any and all sins.

Hanging tough on grades is the most unpleasant, but essential, task in teaching. Your grade is an evaluation of their work, and if it is reasonably fair, is a major responsibility for the teacher. Who else will impersonally, critically, and productively evaluate them? Their friends? Their mothers? Their spouses? Themselves? If they can't see that, you probably will never convince them of its value, so you just have to stiff it out and take the nasty comments in the course evaluation at the end of the course.

No doubt about it - the grading of student work is the most boring, grinding, emotionally-draining task in teaching - assuming that you do it with a real sense of responsibility. But if you know that they got what they needed in the form of instruction and direction, had the necessary opportunity to get clarification of the requirements, and sufficient time to do the work, you **have to** grade them fairly, or you will lose control of the course. Let the goof-offs fall where they may, the diligent students deserve your fair and critical grading.

2.2 Teaching Techniques and Methods

Unfortunately, it really is often quite important **how** you teach. This gives a real edge to the teacher who somehow has a personal combination of technique and method that seems to result in successful teaching. It is a fact: some people are good teachers and some are not. My problem is that in my 33 years of teaching I have yet to hear any reliable formula for what the magic technique and/or method is.

One person's method (translate: program) seldom works for anybody else. It may depend highly on that person's technique (translate: style). The two cannot be separated and you can't use someone else's method if it takes a style that you just don't have the personal characteristics to carry off.

I am not aware of having any particular technique or method, but I surely do. And if it works (as I think it sometimes does), I don't know exactly why.

I try to measure the success of a course by what I judge the students to have accomplished at the end. If most of them passed the final exam; if most of them did a bangup job on the last assignment; etc. - I consider the course a success, even though I might not have done all I had planned to do.

I have had semesters when I thought I did a really great job and everything seemed to go right, and then the end fell apart. I have also had semesters when I thought I really lost the ball and blew the game, only to have the students tell me what a great time they had and how much they learned. It is maddening.

A fundamental problem is that there is a difference between teaching and learning. Teaching is what **you** are doing; learning is what the **students** (hopefully) are doing. You can teach your little heart out, but learning won't happen unless you do some things to try to make it happen.

A lot of teachers make the mistake of thinking that their lectures are the most important part of a course. They stand on this idea in the face of the overwhelming conclusion made by many generations of education researchers that lecturing (somebody talking and everybody else only listening) is the absolutely most **ineffective** means of communication and results in the least retention by the students.

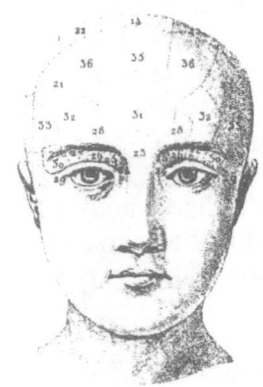

6

If it is mostly all you've got (a lecture course with 300 students), you will have to settle for it. But if there are any opportunities for involving the students more actively, you must take advantage of them. My attitude is that the less I do, and the more the students do, the better for learning. (And, actually, the easier for teaching!)

You may be getting some clues as to my teaching methods. If you want to see my technique, however, you will have to attend my classes. You may think - on an intellectual level - that my methods sound great (or not), but **how** I do it is not separable from the paper work.

2.3 Learning: Context, Process, Goals, and Objectives

Learning is really mysterious, but it is a natural process that occurs in spite of any of our efforts to avoid or thwart it. And with the information overload of current times, we all try to develop defense mechanisms against it.

I personally think that learning happens mostly by infusion. That is, if you submerge yourself long enough in a learning environment, you will unavoidably soak some of it up. If you buy that, I suggest that a major task of the teacher is to provide a learning environment to the extent possible. Coerce the students into attending class and taking part in class activities, provide them with study materials, keep them on their toes with frequent assignments and/or short quizzes, give them rapid feedback on their work. And - at all times - try to see that they have the necessary resources at hand, know exactly what you want from them, and keep up a steady pace of work.

An important factor in learning is context. Teachers tend to focus on their individual courses in a vacuum. Students mostly take several courses at a time, take them in semester sequences, and are caught up in some kind of stream of work (curriculum). It is critical that individual teachers understand this and relate their courses to the students' other current involvements, past experiences, and any expectations from this course for future application. It seems self-evident, but is so often not existent, that it bears emphasizing.

Another context factor is the students' general orientation. For architecture students, this is generally an ambition to be architects; whatever vague, naive image they have of what that means. For the present, because of the strong influence of their design studios, it seems to be a need to design. Anything else you try to make them do that does not have some design context will be compartmentalized by them into a totally separate (and probably inconsequential) activity. And their studio teachers will often reinforce this attitude. That leaves you nothing but the fear factor to use to keep them going.

The learning process in college, unfortunately, is not much different than that in high school. The students are forced to attend class; are made to take particular classes; and are given a defined amount of work - which they will do (if you are lucky) and no more. In other words it is **your** course and curriculum, not their's. It would be nice to try to get them beyond that, but few teachers have succeeded. If you want to try, I still suggest you first give them a firm schedule, clear assignments, and hard due dates. Then go for some inspired effort.

Goals are like the Ten Commandments or the Preamble to the Constitution. It is nice to have some, and every course, curriculum, and school should have them. Keep them few and simply stated, but be sure you know what they are - for both you (the course) and the students (their degree program).

Goals should be reasonably idealistic in character. "To know something about building construction", for example. Objectives should be more specific, pragmatic, and clearly defined. "To know the definitions of all the terms in the Glossary of the course text", for example. Goals address the big picture. Objectives should give you and the students something real to do. Hopefully, performing what is necessary to fulfill the objectives will automatically achieve the goals.

2.4 Communication

Teachers deliver a lecture, make it through the planned topic coverage indicated by their notes, score all the major points brilliantly, and check that one off. Now the students know that! **Right? Not really!**

Communication, especially of ideas and concepts, is hard to achieve and harder to verify. By the time you give the next exam, and find out they missed it all, it is too late to go back and do it all over. Some kind of rapid feedback is necessary. The quick, short assignment; quickly graded and returned is one such device. Short, daily or weekly quizzes are another. The necessity - however accomplished - is to get some indication of whether what you said, or assigned them to read, really stuck with them. Soon enough to repair the damage effectively.

Repetition of major points - to the edge of boredom - is really necessary to burn them in. Quick summaries of the points made in the last lecture should precede the next lecture, if it builds on the last one. Texts should do the same, but not all do. Many authors write and proof-read their own work in a single flow, assuming others will also. Nobody - I mean **nobody** - reads a technical book like a novel; except the author, his editors, and maybe some relentless reviewers.

Communication is more easily tested on a running basis with a small group of students, if they are continuously engaged by questions and discussions. The larger the group, and the more formal the lecture organization, the harder the testing of the effectiveness of the communication you hope is happening. In the latter case, it is really essential to use frequent quizzes or other devices to test the communication.

In this regard, I consider all quizzes and exams to be primarily major testing devices for the effectiveness of the communications. And thus to be real **learning** experiences for both the students and the teacher. The teacher is saying "Here is what I thought you should have learned." And from the test results, the students say "Here is what we didn't get or couldn't handle." Maybe they were goofing off. But just **maybe**, you didn't really get it across.

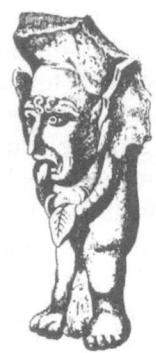

2.5 Learning Progress: Testing and Evaluation

A goal for any course of instruction should be to move the students from some point of lesser knowledge or skill to a higher one. The real achievement of this requires some testing for measurement of the accomplishment. Traditional testing means are with assignments (homework), written exams or quizzes (short, single-question exams), oral exams (questions specifically addressed to selected students in the classroom), personal interviews, and juried presentations of student work.

Just as the lectures and assignments should have specific objectives, so should any evaluation made of tests. Evaluations may be critical for the express purpose of reinforcement or clarification of crucial material. Grading for score achievement is a separate issue. I like to be able to reserve that judgement as a serious issue until all the work is in for the course, and to use all the interim testing for positive purposes as much as possible.

Keep in mind that evaluation of the student's performance is also to some extent a test of the effectiveness of the teaching. If almost **everybody** flunks an exam, there just might have been some lack of effective communication or a general failure of the teaching effort. If nobody in the class seems able to do an assignment, it is probably not really fairly written in relation to your preparation of the students. Give them the benefit of the doubt, and then nail them if you think they really are goofing off and deserve it.

It is essential to be sure that some learning is actually in progress. It is also crucial to try to judge the pace at which you expect it to occur. With a defined time (the semester, etc.) to achieve your purposes, some control of the pace of your's and the students' work is essential.

The best laid plans, however, often go awry, and you should use some testing early on to see if you are going too fast or too slow. And leave some possibilities in the course schedule for slowing down or picking up the pace to respond to your observation of the students' response. The same course, taught in the same curricular spot, may have different results with a different group of students.

Architecture students, especially, tend to have some group dynamic as they form a cloistered group in their program. As a result, there is often some general group character: rebellious, over-achieving, happy and slow, etc. However, you should resist consideration of individual students in this regard. Let them shine in a generally slow group; or have their individual troubles in an over-achieving one.

I personally hate grading curves. I think they are mostly a cop-out for bad teaching, and interfere with the handling of student's individual problems. Admit your mistakes and compensate for them; but hold to some definite achievement standards.

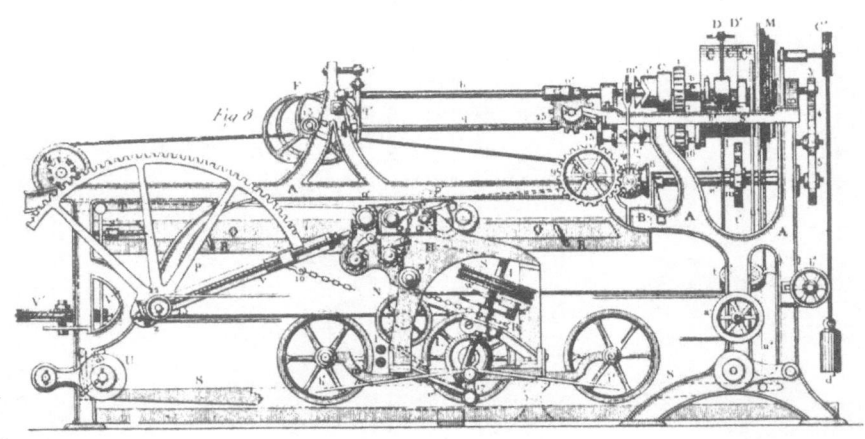

Fig. 8

3

Aids for Teaching and Learning

A principal teaching and learning mechanism is the direct teacher-student contact in the classroom. However, most teachers also use various other devices or methods. This chapter summarizes a few of the most common of these that have some applicability to the subject of building construction.

3.1 Texts

Books for teaching building construction exist in great number, although most tend to facilitate some particular group of students (level, interest, goals, etc.) and all have some limitations. For architecture students (not draftspersons, not spec writers, not estimators, not construction managers, etc.) there are a few that cover the general area of building construction with a broad enough scope to be used as general texts. My current two favorites are:

Fundamentals of Building Construction: Materials and Methods, 2nd edition, by Edward Allen, Wiley, 1991.
Construction Materials and Processes, 3rd edition, by Don Watson, McGraw-Hill, 1986.

Both of these are broad enough in scope to function as texts. Allen's book is profusely illustrated, with many photos and drawings of construction in progress, truly illuminating the process or method, as well as the materials and finished products. Watson's book is organized with the same 16-part Masterformat system as used in **Sweets Catalog Files**, **Architectural Graphic Standards**, and the general construction business. I have used both Allen's and Watson's books as texts for construction courses at different times with reasonable success.

For a traditional course or course sequence in construction materials and methods, either of these books - or several others - may serve well as a course text. My book is intended primarily for a different approach; one that does not aim to blanket the topic of building construction, but rather to favor a point of view that emerges from the building design process.

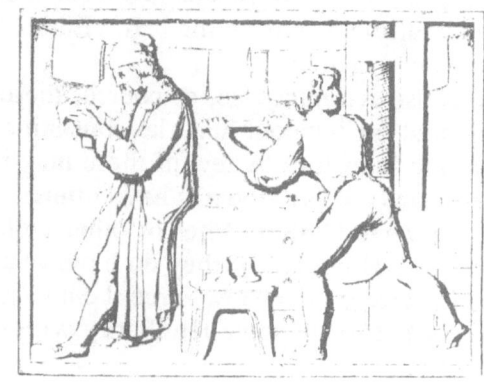

I have hardly ever taught a course without resorting to some kind of supplementary references, outside readings, or other devices to extend the text for the course. Even when it is my text. This book (**Building Construction and Design**) is intended to work with such supplements, and I encourage teachers to consider their use.

I also encourage the use of something to break out of the walls of the classroom - walking tours around the campus, field trips to construction sites, self-guided field trips (send the students out with a map and some notes about buildings along the route).

It is practical and useful to have a text that both you and the students can use for most of the basic course study. It is especially useful for the students outside the classroom. Remember, most of what you say in the classroom goes straight through their heads, in one ear and out the other - less than 5% retention according to researchers in education. If you can, give them a schedule with text coverage references for each lecture or topic in the course. Assume, if you want to, that they may even read the text before coming to the corresponding lecture. Not likely, but a warm thought.

3.2 Course-Specific Materials

I can't imagine teaching a course with nothing but me, the students, and a text. I almost always have some specific purposes or needs for a course that aren't fully covered by the text. Enter: the class notes or handouts.

For a construction course, of course, there is a vast potential for handout material consisting of ads from the industry. A few of these may be good, especially if the students have limited access to **Sweets Catalog Files** or other collected data sources. However, if they do have access to Sweets, I prefer to somehow force them to go there in order to gain some familiarity with using it.

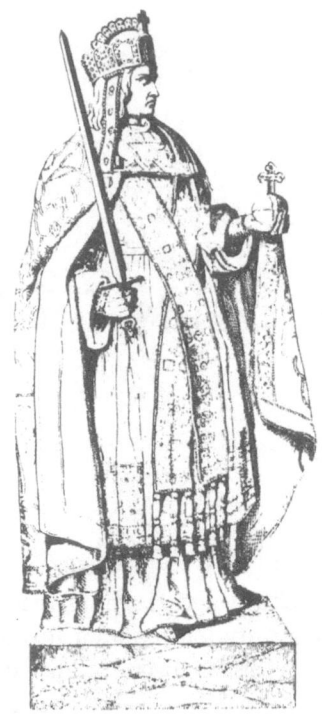

My general experience is that whatever the industry is willing to give you in sufficient number for all the students in a large course is usually not really current and/or of much direct use.

Like me, if the course-specific handouts you need to develop start to exceed the text in mass, it is time for you to write your own text. Welcome to the club of over-worked and under-paid authors.

Try to anticipate the need for any supplements by carefully considering the class sessions and the corresponding text materials. Do this by writing up a schedule that includes actual pages or chapter references for each class period. This should bring to your attention where you have things that you want to do that the text does not provide for. Then you can avoid the mad scramble of trying to get a handout together just before a class. Good advice, but I have at least one mad frenzy with a non-functioning copier in this situation every semester.

Of course, there is a package of materials that are course-specific, consisting of the course syllabus, schedule, assignments, quizzes, and exams. In the best of worlds, you may actually write all of these up before the course begins. Only if you are very weird.

3.3   References and Data Bases

Building construction is a topic for which it is absolutely essential that students develop some experience with the use of available reference sources. These include those in the school library, but more importantly, those that they will primarily access in professional design work. Most likely, they may not then have access to a good library for their purposes.

I cannot imagine coming out of a construction course without having gained some familiarity with Sweets, Ramsey & Sleeper, and some building code. What architecture students need to go forth from their formal construction course work with is some training in how to pursue information on their own; without you, some decaying text, or a canned course package.

And in today's working environment, they should hopefully begin to learn about computer-accessible data bases. Sweets is already available in that form. In professional design offices, operating out of their CAD systems will surely be the normal path for enquiry in any design work in a short time.

Don't worry about exposing them to every nook and cranny of the construction world. Neither you nor they can ever fully treat that. But try to give them some idea of what is out there and how they have to go about using it. Then - if you can - make **them** do the searching on some assignment. Let them experience the world of unintelligible generic language, elusive facts among the advertising hype and hogwash, and all the rest. Dry their tears, but make them suffer the slings and arrows. High school is over.

3.4   Visual Aids

My principal visual aid is a blackboard. I usually fill it with sketches during a lecture. It is hard for me to lecture without one.

My second visual aid is the course text; assuming it is well illustrated. Encourage them to bring it to class and frequently refer to illustrations in it. But be practical - give the page numbers and other data for those who need to look them up later. Other than encouraging them to buy and use the text (for sake of my royalties), this can save you a lot of drawing on the blackboard.

Slides, movies, and videos are entertaining, and can sometimes be impressive and even informative. There are enough available to fill a course schedule, if you want to. I occasionally use them, or provide for visiting lecturers who may use them. But I have come to use them less and less over the years; more or less in inverse proportion to their number and availability. They may be more entertaining than your boring personage in front of the class, but my general experience is that they deliver little per class time expended.

If I use visual aids at all, it is to illustrate something that is otherwise hard to show the students. Such as an earthquake effect produced on a shaking table or some construction sequence in time lapse filming. Of course, slides from your own collection may be regularly used for supplementing the text illustrations and giving some immediate reality to class reading.

If field trips are not possible, some slides or movies may be a second best substitute. Or, you may give a slide show before a field trip to give them the general picture of what they are going out to see and point out things they should pay attention to.

If you must use visual aids, I suggest doing it in class sessions that are otherwise not critical to the flow of the course work. Right after, rather than right before, a big assignment or exam, for example. Maybe in that period at the end of the semester in all architecture schools when they are brain dead from the charrette in their design studios. Give them a break and yourself an easy day.

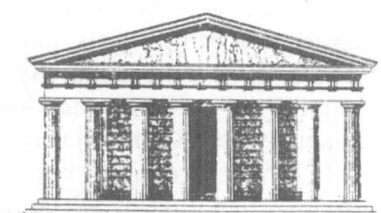

3.5 Samples

I think it is very useful to let students see and handle some real construction materials and products. Some of them will have had a lot of construction experience and it will be a waste of time, but many may have never actually seen or held a piece of gypsum drywall or a joist hanger. I carry what I can into the classroom and let them look and feel if they want to.

There is a spectrum here, from the Bauhaus approach of having them work with the craftspersons and really get physically involved, to relying mostly on books and visual aids. I use what I can to get them into contact with real construction materials and products and the building in progress of construction. The logistics for a large lecture class are troublesome in this regard.

Need for this must relate to any displayed materials that are in the school and to the possibilities for utilizing observations of actual construction in the field.

3.6 Field Observations and Experiences

Most campuses have some construction going on at any given time, so there is a resource available at most times. If you can, walk around the campus once in awhile and give them a report on what is happening that they ought to go and take a look at.

I feel there is a spectrum of exposure here that runs a gamut of effectiveness ranging from the least to the most effective. At the least end is oral or text description of materials and details. At the other end is having them actually build a building. Feasibility of resources and logistics will place you somewhere in this spectrum.

Off-campus field trips are great, but hard to arrange within the scheduling of a lecture course.

If you are teaching a studio, or the students are mostly all in a particular studio while taking your course, you may be able to tag your kind of field trip onto a studio field trip, which is generally more feasible to organize.

While actual visits to construction sites are the best experience, there are substitutes of various kinds. Slide shows and movies may be used for this. Selection of texts or class handouts may be done to fill in for some of this experience. A text with a lot of photos of actual construction in progress (such as Allen's) may be more valuable where field experiences cannot be developed within the course.

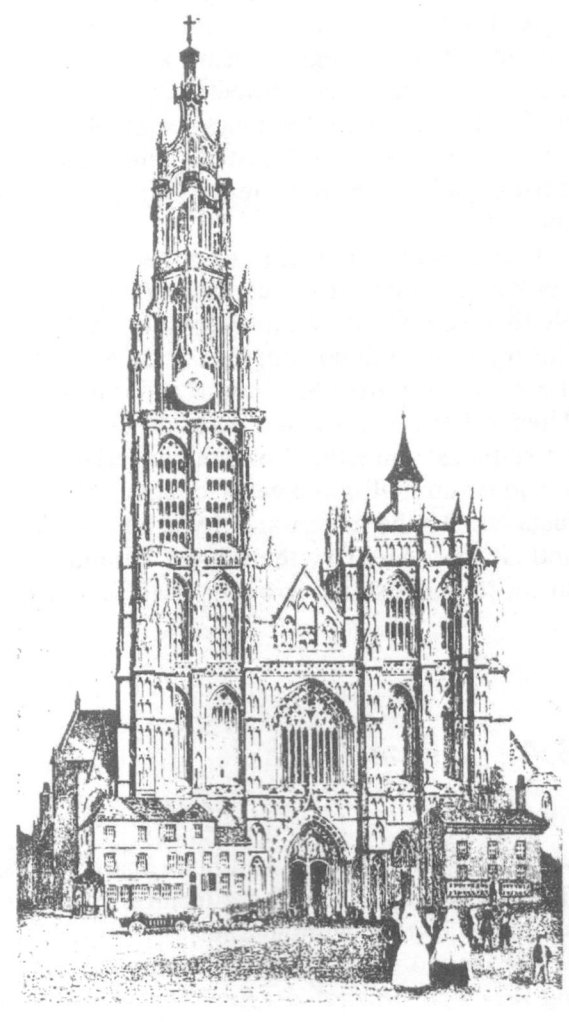

4

Construction as a Study Subject

The following comments are directed at the specific task of teaching about building construction. The orientation here is that of viewing construction as part of the general design problem. Development of construction through choices of materials and systems and working out of construction details is part of the sequence of tasks for building design.

4.1 Existing and Emergent Technologies (The Inventory)

For ease of reference here, I will coin a phrase: The Inventory. This refers generally to what is available at any given time for achieving building construction. It refers to materials, products, systems, processes, and the obtainable output of builders and crafts people.

Utilization of The Inventory for a specific application has somewhat to do with place. The building industry is diffuse, but some materials and systems are more extensively used in particular regions. This may be a matter of provincial customs, but is also a practical issue of simple economic competitiveness and actual availability in some cases.

I assume that what you want to teach is not just what is done in the region or location of the school you are teaching in. However, what the students have opportunities to see, and what local builders and designers do is highly flavored in this regard. Field trips and local visiting lecturers will further burn this in.

In any event, students as designers must be made aware of the continuously changing nature of The Inventory, as well as its range at any given time. But they should also be made to understand that dealing with it once they are out of school means a continuous race to keep up with the changes that occur. This is not a timeless body of knowledge, like plane geometry, to be absorbed once and for all.

My book attempts to give some impression of the potential range of The Technology and often refers to the concept of continuous change. However, the publication process means that the illustrations and any data are frozen in time, and some allowance may have to be made for new issues, new materials, and new design or construction trends.

4.2 History of Technology

My book does not deal much with history. However, much of what we build with is very historically derived or inherited. Most of The Inventory is in some continuous mode of refinement and substitution. Better ways of connecting, sealing, finishing, protecting, and doing many things are discovered and absorbed into The Inventory.

We now use mortars better than our ancestors dreamed of. But we hardly ever make stone masonry with structural stone masonry units. We use CMUs, stone veneers, imitative composites, and a lot of things to make something resembling stone masonry, but we just don't lay up stones in mortar much any more.

Much of what we do today will in a very short time be viewed as historical and quaint. Our students will discard what we use and find new ways - maybe better, maybe not. Some attention to history should be used to emphasize this ongoing changing nature of The Inventory.

In my book I attempt to describe basic construction concepts in a way that relates to fundamental needs and issues and try not to dwell on what is the right way to build at any particular time. Whatever the right way is at the moment, it won't be right a short time from now. But the basic needs will go on: keep the water from coming through the roof; the paint from peeling off the walls; the floors from squeaking; the pipes from sweating; and the doors from sticking shut. And do it all intelligently with The Inventory that exists at the moment in time that the work occurs.

4.3 Finding Out About Construction

A major problem for all of us - students, teachers, authors, design practitioners - is simply finding out what is in The Inventory at any given time. It constitutes an immense collection of data and is not very fully ordered for our educational, discovery, or design purposes. The information systems that exist are primarily oriented to the selling of products and services, keeping accounts, regulating the construction, and writing specifications.

Students need to be made to accept that what you can tell them, or any text can show them, is very limited in scope. There is a lot more information available, but they have to gain experience in how to get to it and how to deal with the sales hype and the general data overload.

I consider this a critical concern, and my approach in the book is to try to show that the students must accept that it is **their** problem to go after information, just to learn how to chase it down. If they are going to be building designers, they will be in the chase for life and the sooner they understand how it works and what the problems are in it, the better for their design education.

For doing class assignments, they and you will probably have to accept the limitations of available resources: starting with you, the text, the school library, etc. But they should see that for professional work, they won't be excused from being fully aware of The Inventory.

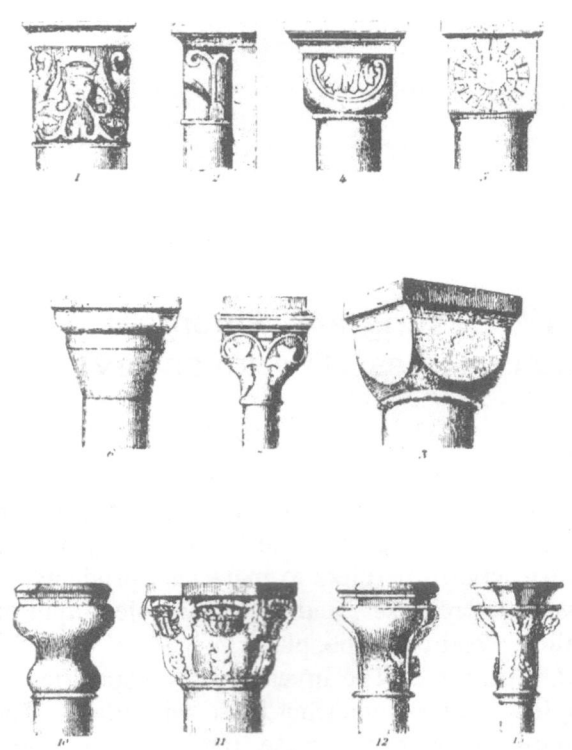

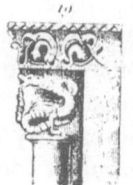 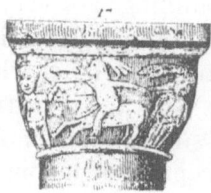 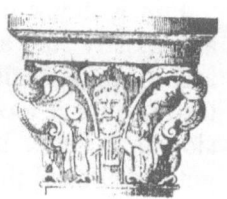 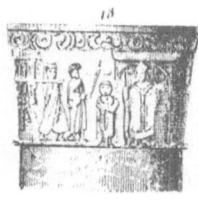 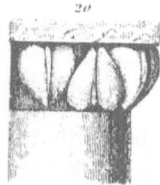 

What tends to be the easiest to find out, of course, is the most common way of doing things. The current "way" of doing things gets to be that by a lot of really pragmatic considerations. But the potential for variation in any situation is enormous. My book mostly concentrates on illustrative examples that are deliberately quite common in nature. This leaves the door open to bring in endless examples of other, possibly more interesting, maybe better ways of doing things.

My general method is to explain the basic problems and issues in a situation; then show the time-tested response; and then more-or-less challenge the students to look for other ways besides the common one. I don't accept that the common solutions are automatically to be rejected. But what is commonly done is not always so because it is the best in all regards. Most likely it is the cheapest, the easiest, the most successfully marketed, and the most familiar to everybody in the industry. But its performance is surely not best in some regards; maybe not in hardly any that have real design value.

I feel that looking for better ways has to be done with the common way known first, so that going beyond it is a conscious effort. The students have to expect to have their designs compared to the common ways, and they should be able to defend their work with this reference frame.

4.4 Using the Construction Inventory

Making use of the full range of The Inventory for design work is fraught with many difficulties. My book treats this issue and refers to it often, since I think it needs to be clearly understood.

The sheer mass of information, its constantly changing nature, the form of most information (sales hype, prejudiced viewpoint, etc.), and any individual's capacity for collating it are all factors in creating this problem.

Still, any real design work has to be achieved by coping with the situation. This is a place where some examples of personal experience from a teacher's own design work may be very useful. Or, possibly, some case studies from books or magazines or from visiting lecturers. How were the alternatives (in terms of construction materials and systems) considered in the design process?

A problem here is that "design presentations" in books, magazines, exhibits, and star lectures seldom contain much detail about the construction. A sad reason for this is that "designers" sometimes don't care about or simply don't know much about construction.

I truly believe that this is an area where the computer age will bring some real accomplishments. The ability to access, scan, evaluate, and test enormous amounts of information with computer-stored data bases and computer-aided design processes makes it feasible to consider a much larger part of The Inventory for a single application then ever before. Development of the designer's awareness still needs to be dealt with, but the handling of mass data and the comparative analysis of alternatives using real facts should be within reach. If you believe in informed design, this is cause for rejoicing.

There are, I am told, human beings who are capable of memorizing the entire Encyclopedia Britannica. For my part, after some 50 years of involvement in construction, I still discover something new every week. And I think when I can't find anything new any more, I will wrap the drapery of my couch about me and lie down to pleasant dreams.

4.5 Creating (Designing) Construction

Construction for most buildings is not so much designed as it is simply assembled like a collage from bits and pieces of familiar elements. Every imaginable element is cataloged and numbered by the CSI, whose wildest dream is that the time will come when "drawings" can be totally disposed with, and the construction can be fully described by a numerically coded bit map in the computer. With each code number referring to a beautifully written specification in the CSI Master Library.

If you think this is an Orwellian nightmare fantasy, you haven't been involved with the CSI lately. In case you haven't noticed, the CSI is emerging as the key group in the organization of the construction industry. Architects still make "presentations", but the CSI documents it all in excruciatingly organized detail. The general "look" of buildings may be an architectural decision, but the specific ingredients, quality, and finish of the construction are in the specifications, and the control is in the hands of the writer (and selector) of the specs.

Designing of construction (not just assembling coded, canned elements) means working from basic concepts to produce original solutions. That takes several things:

Full understanding of the basic concepts.

Familiarity with current technology (The Inventory), sufficient to use it for your particular -   and maybe unique - purposes.

Ability to use normal channels (construction drawings and specifications) to transmit your design to the run of the mill people who will actually execute the work.

Ability to defend your work in response to standard questions: Will it work? How much will it cost? How long will it take? What is better about it than the good old way of doing things? Can you really be sure what will happen as it ages, gets rained on, freezes, the sun beats down on it, and time generally goes by?

Fun is fun, but buildings are very expensive and mostly stay around for a long time. The architectural decisions may be capriciously made (how weird it looks), but the construction decisions had better be soundly made. You can toy with the visual perception of it, but you can't fool mother nature.

Exciting, meaningful, lasting innovations are mostly done by designers who are either just lucky or who (more likely) work very hard and who apply some genius to the work.

I really don't think the CSI will ever take over the collating of the coded elements into whole buildings. Architects may have increasingly less influence on what the elements are, but the collating will always be an architectural task, and the people who do it will be architects, whatever names they travel under. An architect is an architect is an architect.

All the more to view building construction as an **architectural** problem, which is hopefully primarily what my book is about. Give The Technology due acknowledgement for its existence, accept that it changes continuously and maybe you can nudge the change a little, and let the spec-writers do what they do best - write good specifications. All's well that ends well!

4.6 Evaluating Designs

How indeed can a particular construction design be evaluated? Well, that depends on the value references. If you only mean "How does it look?", the answer is a very personal and subjective one and pretty much off the computer. And not much dealt with in my book. If you mean "How much does it cost?", "How long will it take?", "How does it compare to the usual way of doing things?", and other hard, quantifiable questions, you have to meet the Value Analyst and be introduced to the world of Value Analysis or Value Engineering.

Value analysis is a basic ingredient of fundamental systems design and has been around a long time for some folks who have been using systems design concepts and processes extensively since

18

the earliest days of the computer. In the fields of product design, military hardware, political science, economics, and hazard mitigation this is routine stuff. In architecture it is pretty much a frontier.

For educational purposes we can go at this in a single item-by-item manner and make some token analyses just to show the process. In real design work, it had better be done with an intelligent procedure and the best of accessible facts. Take any of the details in the nine case study buildings in Chapter Ten of my book and pose the question:

"How can we do this better to improve the _____?

You fill in the blank. Cost. Look. Water resistance. Thermal response. Ease of construction.

Give it a shot with some examples. Or let the students try. Make them come up with some facts to prove their point, if you think they can. It is a very useful exercise.

4.7 Design-Oriented Studies

I think that there are many aspects of the subject of construction that designers need to be aware of. It becomes - for practical reasons - a matter of how much and what kind of knowledge is required. Is it enough to be generally aware and somewhat familiar with some aspect, or is truly professional-level, operative skill a necessity?

Building designers surely ought to know something about basic materials and their production, manufacturing processes, determination of costs for estimates, management of the construction work, the general nature and functions of contracts, and the problems of writing good specifications. The more that is known about all these things, the better grip that can be had on the whole of the subject and its relations to design.

But what is at the heart of the designer's responsibility is the need to **design**. This means that the approach to any subject that impinges on design work must eventually be made from inside the design process. What do I really have to know about construction in order to do intelligent design? To the extent that this approach can be taken, I have tried to take it in developing my book.

I see this design-oriented approach as posing two questions that should be considered in any design decision.

1. How might consideration of construction problems affect or limit a basic architectural design decision regarding plan form, exterior detail, scale, etc.?

2. How might a design decision - made for purely architectural design reasons - generate construction problems? For example, what construction problems are created by having a particular roof shape, a certain magnitude of span, or a form of exterior detail?

Design development means making these analyses again and again. It may be done by "hand", as in the good old days. Or it may be done with a computer-aided procedure, bought in a package or developed by you. If you can't ask and answer the questions to yourself, they will be asked by others, and the answering and the decisions about how to respond may be taken out of your hands.

The meanest part of value analysis is defining the values and quantifying them or ordering their priorities. What is more important? Cost? Safety? Code compliance? Energy conservation? Construction time? What exactly does "best" mean? It is scary to contemplate a building design process where the architect is not operatively involved in this analysis process, but rather just waits in the reception room while the jury deliberates.

This is really an extremely important and sensitive issue in contemporary design practice. Constructive criticism of design is the single most important ingredient in teaching design. It will always be some mixture of subjective and objective analyses, but the fact-based analysis is becoming increasingly a demand by the world outside the architectural design studio.

19

5

The Professional Designer

Before proceeding with the chapters on teaching work itself, I would like to delve a bit deeper into my views about the working context of the professional building designer. My book is developed from this background, so it may be helpful for the user to know what peculiar attitudes have flavored the work.

5.1 Working Context

Most designers today work in some kind of team design situation. This is organizationally structured if they are in a large design firm, but it also happens even if they are single practitioners running a one-person office. Modern buildings and their designs, and the organization of the construction business are too complex to allow for the lone operator of design.

Somebody on the design team has the command decision role; sometimes called the **prime designer**, although they may not really be a "designer" at all, but basically a management person. All of this still leaves the building designer (project architect, etc.) to do the design development work, but it must happen in some kind of reviewed situation.

Continuous reviews come from the other members of the design team as the work progresses. Staged, scheduled, major reviews come at significant times, relating to the overall progress and approval of the work by someone with command decision authority. Maybe by the persons who are paying for it all.

Design of large and/or complex buildings takes a long time, and there has to be some real progress in the design development. Hopefully the reviews do not always result in a lot of backtracking and rerunning of the same routines to get different solutions; otherwise progress may never really occur.

Design methodologies and operative procedures must function to allow some rational and effective progress of the design work - without, hopefully, totally squelching the creative spirit of the right-brain dominated designer. For some systemized development, the procedures also need to facilitate two things:

Some ongoing exchange between the designer and the rest of the people involved in the work (other designers; consultants in general; the boss; the draftspersons; etc.). The simple inquiry, "how's it going?", should be met with an immediate documented response.

Some ongoing anticipation of review (judgment, jury, approval, reconsideration, office cash flow analysis, etc.).

This means that the design should be continuously documented in some form of display that is readable by others without much help. It should also be reaching, of sorts. That is, it should be up to the minute with the firm decisions, but include some speculative versions (sketches) of what needs yet to be done, but is not quite firmed up.

In my own practice (in theory; in the best of times and circumstances) I endeavored to keep an ongoing-developed set of drawings of the work; displayed at two levels. Everything reasonably fully developed was displayed in finished detail. Everything else was in sketch form. The combination presented as complete a picture as we could visualize. Some of it was still fuzzy, but at least defined in some understandable display.

For the development of the construction design, this meant basically working up the scale in terms of drawings. As soon as the basic form of the building was worked out (1/16th inch plans and elevations, say), we would draw up the complete plans, elevations, and some full-building sections at that small scale. From those full-building sections, then, we could essentially define all the detailed working sections that needed definition in highly detailed fashion to fully describe the construction.

Then we steadily increased the size of the drawings, as specific detail choices, material choices, and specification writing proceeded. At all times - and maybe even at the end for the construction drawings - we kept the whole set together. Thus, someone could first scan the small scale drawings and get the big picture; move to the next scale and see in more detail some units, such as whole wall sections in some detail; and finally see the detailed construction with notation at as large a scale as necessary for a complete understanding (by you and the builder).

This is actually the basic rationale for the displays in the case studies in Chapter Ten of my book. For each case, the first display is a set of very small, but mostly whole-building, drawings - to get the big picture. Then some more detailed drawings of significant units. And finally, if necessary (as for the curtain walls in some examples), larger details of single elements.

In this regard, each of the case studies in Chapter Ten may be visualized as displaying a design at some intermediate stage; with the big picture defined and some of the typical construction developed to a degree. For teaching, or for a student assignment, you could pick up any of these cases and finish it; redo it better; modify it to change some particular performance - cost, energy conservation; bring it into conformance with some selected building code, etc.

Whether done in my style and personal graphic technique (freehand, marker sketches over blue-line drafted layouts; basically for photo-reproduction, so the blue lines fade out in the copies), or in some other media - maybe a CAD system, this is generally how design work proceeds. Not in a smooth, linear fashion, of course. Some details may actually be worked out first in some cases. But, somehow, the whole picture, and the whole job, must be kept in view as the detailed development proceeds to the necessary level of completion.

Anyway, that process is what I assume the typical designer to be involved in while confronting the need to know something about construction. And that is how I tried to develop the book; to view the topic from that situation.

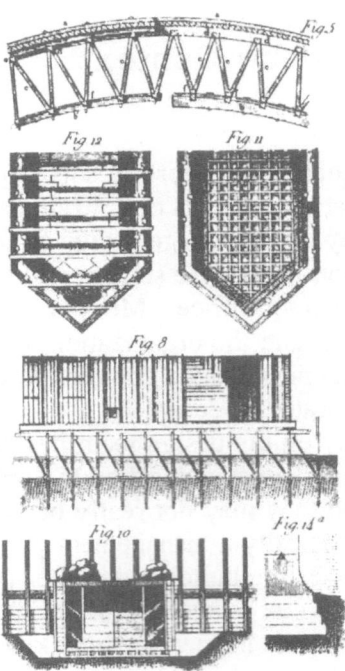

5.2 Professional Liability

The recent situation with increasing nastiness regarding liability is one reason I decided to get out of professional practice. Others, I hope, are enduring and the profession goes on; I am happy in other endeavors. The more designers work to do some creative design of construction, the more personal responsibility they take on. If they do everything regarding construction in the good old ways (material usage, standard products designed by someone else, tried-and-true details), they dodge professional liability as much as possible.

In this climate, it is naive and irresponsible to pressure students to think creatively without making them understand the potential consequences. You don't want to scare them out of trying to become architects, but I think you need to keep close to reality somehow.

My personal attitude is that I think it is possible to create some great architecture without having necessarily to reinvent the whole building process and The Inventory every time you design a building. Thank God for those who push the frontiers with new concepts and innovative methods in construction, but architecture is a lot more than just construction. I think a great designer could conceivably outshine the Taj Mahal with gypsum drywall, stud construction, and EFI cladding. Just as a really great photographer could probably produce some winning art with the cheapest K-Mart camera. The media doesn't have to be the message.

One more reason for using The Inventory in its simplest forms to illustrate basic construction issues and problems. Why not show the easiest, most accepted, most time-tested way of doing it first? Then if you can, pick it apart for good cause and show some more inspired or demonstrably better ways of doing it.

5.3 Contracts

I am not a lawyer, but I have signed a lot of contracts, written a few, testified in court, and served on juries. Most building designers work within a relationship defined somehow by a legal contract. Besides the issue of professional liability (and having your children's inheritance paid out in lawyers' fees), the contract that covers the design work probably also spells out where the designer's responsibilities start and end. If it doesn't, there are some general statutes or precedents that imply the limits to some degree.

Hopefully, designers are not responsible for the basic properties of materials or for the reliability and performance of manufactured products. However, they probably are responsible for picking basic materials and products for appropriate uses and showing people what those uses are. They are also hopefully not responsible for the builders' work. But they are, probably, responsible for telling a builder to do something that is stupid, even though they ought to know it is stupid and not do it.

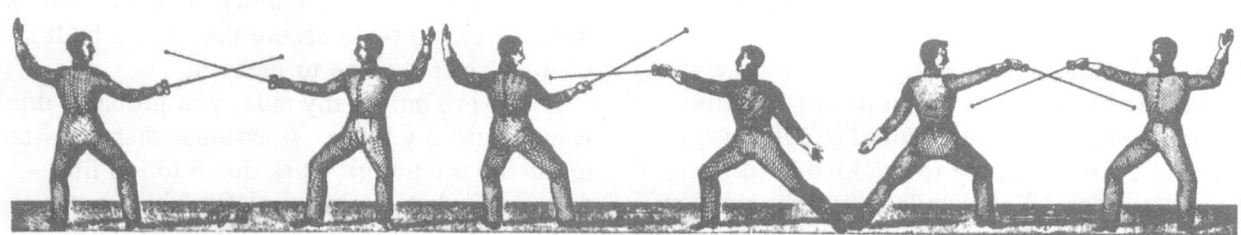

23

Although I did it a lot in my youth, I wouldn't do any design work now without having all this clearly established. Especially if it was innovative in the slightest way regarding construction. All the other parties in the building business are very, very careful with contracts, and it behooves the designer to be also. A very large number of lawsuits against architects have to do with the nonperformance of some detail of a building's construction. Water leakage leading the pack.

Whether to really worry the students in a construction course about all of this depends somewhat on their level in the curriculum. Don't scare beginning students too much with it, but give it some discussion with upper level or graduate students. You won't have to worry about bringing it up with people who are out of school and working; they are probably already in the middle of one lawsuit or another and will bring it up themselves.

5.4 Working Drawings

Construction drawings, or working drawings as we used to call them, are the primary transmittal of the architect's design to those who will bring it into physical existence. The critical role of the specifications notwithstanding, the drawings really define the building design.

Teaching about construction (the physical reality of buildings) has to relate somewhere to how architects themselves deal with construction. They don't do the building work; they don't even much write the specifications; but they do make the working drawings. In a curriculum that does not include separate courses on making working drawings, I think the construction courses need to deal with some of the problems of making working drawings.

My book is not about making working drawings, but it is about construction from an architect's viewpoint. And thus a lot of the illustrations are in a form relating to the kind used for working drawings. The detailed cut section being a major primary element.

The cut section is highly useful in explaining the guts of construction. Not the finished look, but how it goes together. It appears a lot on working drawings for good reasons. And it ought to show up a lot in a construction course. And the students ought to be made to draw some themselves. Not just for the drafting exercise, but that doesn't hurt either.

5.5 Specifications

I don't write contracts anymore, I let lawyers do it. It doesn't mean that I don't read them or try to understand them; I just think others can write than better than I can.

I also don't much write specifications anymore, I let the CSI or somebody else do it. Same reasons.

Designers mostly dodge any contact with specs. Unfortunately, that also usually includes ever reading them or trying in the least to understand them. They thus lose effective control over the finished quality of their constructed work. It may **look** like what they designed, but that's it.

Of course, that may be all they really care about: how it looks for the professional photographer right after it is finished. In which case, they have no need whatsoever for my book. Some very famous designers have expressed such a view, and I think their work speaks for itself.

I don't think that is the general case. For me, personally, I don't really believe that construction is the be-all and end-all of architecture, but I do think it is important to try to control it a bit. So I try to work it out with the limits of my abilities; draw it as clearly as I can; read the specs (whoever wrote them); and generally be as involved as I think I need to be to assure that it gets built as well as I can manage to make it.

If you are not on my side, you probably don't want to use my book. It assumes that you want to pursue the design work down to the final degree of what it takes to define the construction adequately.

5.6 Economics

A major concern for building construction is its cost. Clients are generally much more concerned about this than about whether the bricks are exactly the right shade of pink. Designers are not quite as concerned about costs, except that they know they are accountable for them to some degree.

Construction costs are only ever truly known when the job is done and the bill is paid. Before that they are mostly somebody's guess; politely called The Estimate. Estimating construction costs is serious business and deserves a lot of attention in professional design practice and in education. It doesn't get its due in either case, mostly, for various reasons. It is just behind water leakage in the number of liability cases.

My book deals very little with economics, except to point it out in some general situations and to explain the reasons why some materials, products, or systems are so popular. Serious treatment of cost estimating requires a major presentation that simply couldn't be included in this book. It shouldn't be ignored, but seems to me to require a whole separate effort (and another book; another course) to be adequately done.

6

Situations for Teaching

This chapter deals with the various possible situations that may occur in which some teaching of construction takes place. And, if I can stretch it, some ideas about how my book can be used for the teaching effort.

6.1 The Architecture Curriculum

Having taught as long as I have, and in three different schools, I have had considerable experience with shaping architecture curricula and the components thereof. NAAB-approved curricula have some relatively common elements and mostly some common forms. Still, there is a lot of room for variation, while still managing to keep the NAAB happy.

Variation is especially wide with regard to the non-studio courses. Some programs have a lot of construction courses; some have - believe it? - none. If there are construction courses, they may be essentially working drawing drafting courses, lecture courses about history, theory, and the romance of construction, or something else.

At the time of this writing, I teach the one and only hard stuff, technology-oriented, construction course in the architecture program in my school.

I teach it to students in their third semester of the ten semester program for the B Arch degree. They have yet to have any other technology courses (structures, HVAC, etc.). This is a context that I feel highly obligated to relate to.

From my experience, it is silly to dream about the perfect architecture curriculum or the perfect course of any kind. As designers, most architecture faculty go on tinkering with the educational program as long as they are in it. Meanwhile, at any given time, you have to relate to the real context with regard to the students in a particular course in a particular semester.

A particular problem is that of the relationship between the architectural design studios and the rest of the curriculum. The studios are both the students' womb to crawl back into and the torture chamber where they expend all their emotions and energy. You get the leftovers in other courses. I have taught both studios and lecture courses, so I have seen it all.

You have to hold your ground regarding the importance of your non-studio course. Otherwise, they will totally abandon you. But you need to be real about their studio commitments. If you haven't bothered to determine the studio schedule, you will surely find out when the big pushes occur in the studios; just look at all the empty seats in your lecture classroom.

More idealistically, it should be a major educational goal to make the separate elements of the curriculum relate to each other. This is clear for sequential courses (Construction 101, 102, etc.), but seldom achieved with the courses for separate topics in the curriculum.

I think in at least half of the semesters in my career somebody has formed a committee to coordinate the studios with the rest of the courses to integrate the curriculum. And it has almost never actually happened.

You are a part of the curriculum. It is around you; it will affect you; and you will affect it. But it is tough to manage some sensible relationship. However, at the least, you should stay aware of the specific current curricular arrangements and the specific content of any related courses that precede or follow yours.

You should also be aware of the full content of the semester program for the students in your course. Is there any way for you to relate what you are doing to what other things they are doing in the same semester or the same week?

6.2 Lecture Courses

Most of the required architecture courses in architecture programs consist of one of two kinds. First is the studio (lab/workshop) in which the principal topic is "design". For accreditation, the student/teacher ratio in these must be kept around 15:1.

Most architecture schools prefer to give individual studio courses a generous space (50 to 75 sq ft per student) and let them use if all the time; not sharing a student's assigned work space with any other course. The combination of low student/teacher ratio and space gobbling makes these very expensive courses. This usually absorbs about 90% of the school's teaching budget (for salaries, rent, equipment, staff support, etc.).

The lecture courses - the other basic form - mostly run to student/teacher ratios of 50:1 or more (I average about 90:1). They meet in short class time (typically 50 minutes/week/credit hour). And they use some fully-shared lecture room; often chasing another class out the previous period and being chased out by one the next period. This does not favor much casual contact

with students before or after class, and further works to characterize the feeling of formality of the lecture class.

If the teacher is lucky, there may be some help from a student assistant for some of the drudgery of handling students and/or class materials. This can be some actual help, or can actually **add** to your work if you have to find things for the TA to do and have to undo some of their work with the students. My experience has been mostly the latter. TA appointments are often a principal device for attracting graduate students (especially in expensive private schools) and appointments do not much relate to actual potential for teaching assistance.

I won't dwell on the studios here. I bring them up just to make the contrast clear between the situations for the studio (the student's loving home base) and the lecture room for the construction course (mob scene, nap time, boredom infinitum). Deducting for start up, shut down, passing out stuff, taking attendance, interruptions for answering stupid questions, etc., a one hour class (actually 50 minutes to start with) leaves you about 25 minutes of lecture time at best. You had better talk fast, have a lot of good notes, draw very quickly on the blackboard (you have your back to the students and can lose control in a few seconds), and maintain the upper hand at all times. Show the slightest chink in your armor, and they will instantly go for the kill.

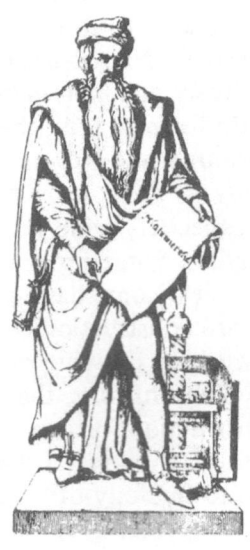

My first semester ever in teaching I had a 1:00 class. I never ate lunch because of my nervous stomach. I lived in mortal dread of finishing up ten minutes before the end of the period with nothing more to say. If I let them go early, they would make noise in the acoustically-awful halls and disturb the rest of the classes. Why I ever stayed around for another semester, I will never know!

Now, I sometimes take a nap before a lecture; often work with no notes at all; and finish early whenever possible. Remember the 5% retention rule, their 10 minute maximum attention span, and your many other career opportunities.

You have to relate to the pragmatic logistics of the course form, student/teacher ratio, lack of any effective assistance, straight jacket of the course schedule (hour of the day, length of the lecture period, class days/week, total lectures/semester). And any other unchangeable facts (bad lecture room, classes preceding you or chasing you out of the lecture room, lecture room on the opposite side of the campus, etc.).

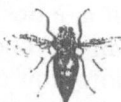

You really **have to** make up a course schedule with the dates for all the lecture topics, assigned readings, exam times, assignment due dates, etc., and stick to it as much as possible. I usually do this on a one page handout, given out at the first class. (See my examples in Chapter 7.) You should share this with the teachers of the studios that your students are taking, and ask for the studio schedule. It won't mean much, because you will change your schedule and the studios will change their's and neither of you will tell the other, but it helps establish a friendly relationship at the outset that will offset the bad ones later when your students do their lecture homework in the studio and sleep in the lecture room during big pushes in the studio.

As I have said before, researchers state that communication delivered in the form of one person talking and a lot of others only listening results in a maximum of about 5% retention. If there is something you really want them to get, you need to say it $1/0.05 = 20$ times; preferably on 20 separate occasions.

I offer the following points for giving lectures on a very technical subject to essentially right-brain, half-awake people.

1. Do not read from your notes. If you want them to know what is in your notes, hand them out or write them on the blackboard.

2. Do not recite in a lecture what is clearly written in the text. Tell them it is in the text; that you expect them to read it and will quiz them on it. Then go on to elaborate on, or to argue with what is in the text. And then quiz them on both the text and your lecture. After a few times of this, they may get the point.

3. Use visual aids, dramatic gestures, back ground sound effects, funny costumes, or - if you have it - a sense of humor to lighten up and break the boredom of your lectures.

My book is not intended as a set of lecture notes. However, it has a lot of materials - both text and graphic - that can be incorporated into a combined attack of lectures and outside reading. In this regard, remember that you only get them for a few minutes a week, but they can eat, sleep, and generally take up housekeeping full time with my book.

If you are going to use a text, make **them** use it. Refer frequently in your lectures to portions of the book, assuming they either have it with them or can look in it after class. Give them page numbers and titles of items.

What you can expect to accomplish with a given set of lectures depends a lot on the number of lectures, length of time for individual lectures, and the total time span for the lecture series. The normal school semester (14 weeks + or -) with two or three lectures per week is a standard form, and the one I generally relate to in this manual.

I teach a 3-credit construction lecture course that meets for two 1.5 hour periods (actually 80 minutes) per week for approximately 14 weeks. I don't count much on the first day and don't expect much from the last two days because of the end-of-the-semester crunch in the studios (mine included).

I also expect to lose about five or six other days to my own exams, unannounced studio field trips, big due dates in the studios, student riots, bomb scares, my illnesses or fully brain-dead (so call in sick) days, etc. That leaves me about 20 real class periods a semester to do the job.

You may have more or less than that. If there is more than one construction course in the curriculum, and there is some real sequence between them, your job may be a fractional part of the whole subject. If you have to incorporate other objectives in the course (spec writing, drafting, cost estimating, etc.), you may have limited time for the basic construction study.

It may be that you do not have a full-fledged course at all. Maybe you are doing a lecture series within a studio, as an extension offering, or in some other situation. I think my book can be used in some of these situations, but it probably needs more than a few lectures to do the whole topic some justice. However, my book is so reader-friendly and entertaining, that I am sure it might be able to carry the momentum from a one-day seminar if the reader gets sufficiently jump-started.

I discuss some of the other course or situation uses besides the full semester course later in this chapter.

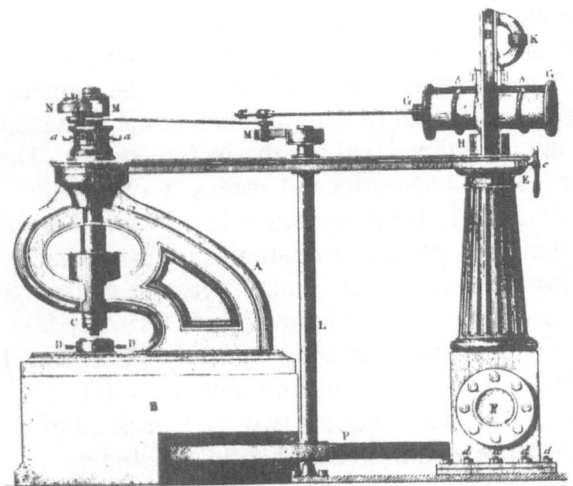

6.3 Lecture/Lab Courses

Although I don't have the luxury of it at present, I think the ideal situation for teaching construction is a lecture/lab situation. By that I mean a combined lecture series that formally develops the whole topic and a lab/workshop/studio adjunct to the lectures. A conceivable alternative would be a studio dedicated to a major involvement in construction with a series of adjunct lectures.

By whatever means, the idea is to have the best of both situations. A deliberately developed lecture series, but with a kind of working situation that permits assignments other than what a large lecture class can logistically handle. "Design" assignments, if you will, with a purpose relating to the lecture-developed materials. The assignments get "crits" on a running basis from the teacher(s).

This arrangement would greatly strengthen the view that construction is a design problem; which is the primary thesis in my book. After a little introductory orientation, you could pose a problem of a design nature, and then go on to use the lectures and workshop crits in tandem to develop the problem assignment.

This kind of offering, of course, cannot be accomplished with a student/teacher ratio of 50:1 or more. It either requires a lot of help from really qualified student assistants or a faculty team to handle a large group. It also requires more scheduled class time and two different teaching spaces: the lecture room and a studio/lab space. For all of these and other reasons, I can't manage it at the moment in my school. But I still think it is the best way to go.

My book can help this kind of course a lot, especially with the case studies as sample forms for an assignment involving the definitive development of an architectural scheme. That is pretty much what the nine examples in Chapter Ten consist of. You wouldn't want the students to just copy those, but you could use one or more as a model for an assignment. I try to do it in a lecture course, but the development of the assignments and the grading is a nightmare.

6.4 Studios

The image of the architectural design studio has a long history and heritage. What happens there is mostly very heuristic and not much subject to any didactic approach in terms of topics or nature of the work. It is magic time; not $1 + 1 = 2$. It is also mostly limited pretty much to dealing with design in what normally constitutes only the preliminary design stages in a professional office; a long way from the final working drawings and specs stage.

It is possible, of course, to have a "studio" that actually involves students beyond the preliminary design phase. Or even one that fully forsakes the preliminary design by essentially starting off with a design from that stage and jumps into the next, more definitive stage. If so, it is conceivable that an adjunct lecture series for such a studio may develop the subject of construction sufficiently in a disciplined way to kill two birds: teach the students something about construction in general, and support the studio assignments.

This is a hard case to sell; mostly because of the long-standing tradition of us and them - the studios and the other courses in architecture schools. Plus the fact that most studio teachers are professionally concentrated on design as traditionally viewed and as typically very slickly presented. They may, in fact, actually not be qualified to teach construction. In any case, it hardly ever happens, so it is either a bad idea or somehow essentially cross grain to the architecture heritage.

As a result, most architecture students never really encounter the necessity to carry design work past the preliminary design stage until they go to work in a professional design office. And then, when they can't, both they and the office bleed profusely.

If ever, anywhere, any time, there is a studio that wants to carry design into the stages where the construction must be developed, I truly think my book can help. It could be used for an adjunct lecture series, or simply be worked with on the assignments. It could be a coalescing reference, from within which extensions can be made to all other available sources: Sweets Files, Architectural Graphic Standards, industry handbooks, etc. A pleasant dream.

6.5 Level (Year) in the Curriculum

Any specific course offering must relate to the particular level of experience of the students. Although teaching techniques, methods, and even the actual teaching materials (texts, visual aids, etc.) may be the same, the presentation, pace, and expectations for a course must relate to the prior, current, and anticipated experiences of the class.

A first or second year course in an architecture program cannot have the same pace or expectations as a fifth year or graduate course. Among other things that the beginning student does not have is a command of the lingo: the special vocabulary, language, jargon, and unique terminology of the field. This may include commonly used words that have different meanings when used in discussing certain things in the field. "Specs", for example, is a common slang word for eye glasses. But to everyone in the construction design and building field it is short for specifications.

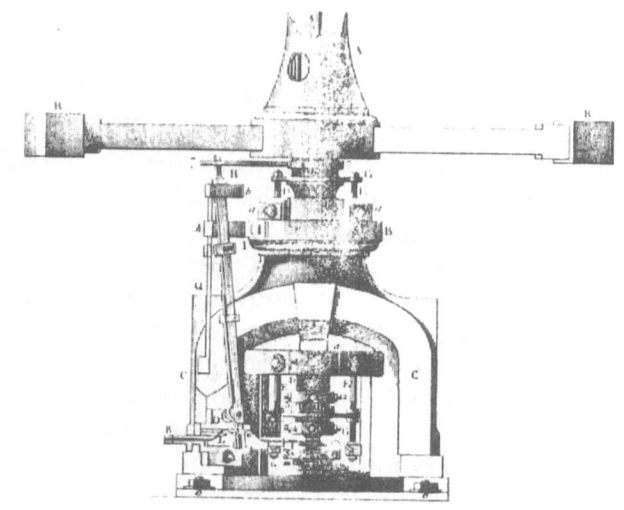

31

I include a glossary (short, specific-purpose dictionary) in almost all of the technical books I write, for two reasons. The first purpose is so that readers can find out exactly what I mean when I use the words in my book. It is really **my** glossary, even though I try to make it correspond to current accepted definitions as much as possible.

The second purpose of the glossary is to provide vocabulary lessons for the reader. When using such a book for a text, I usually have quizzes or exams that test the vocabulary to inspire the students to study. Learning the word meanings helps a little to get into the concepts that the words represent.

A better test, of course, is to use the words in some declarative statement that gets to the context, significance, and association of the words. I test that too, in many cases. Thus, a quiz may test only the recognition of the word and its brief definition; an exam question may ask for interpretation of some declaration that uses the word in a true or false or multiple choice form.

Precise relationships to the level of the student are actually hard to handle. In the first place, in a large class, all the students are not the same in their background experience, even though they may all be second year architecture students. Nor are they all the same in their learning skills or difficulties, basic intelligence, general motivation, maturity, etc. If you work with a single group of students long enough, you have to try to get some handle on the general capacity and needs of the group; but hopefully also handle those who are either way below or way past the general group achievement.

While you may expect some understandable differences between student groups at different levels, you also have to recognize that they are all adults (in college) and also that students are students - no matter the level.

Don't talk down to the first year students. Talk to them like adults, while allowing for their inexperience in terms of prior exposure to the subject. But also expect a class of graduate students - or even mature professionals long out of school - to act like students. They will goof off on the homework, not study for exams, complain about grades, and bring in lame excuses for their short-

comings. In my experience, the group most likely to not meet the deadlines on their homework assignments or design projects are the graduate students; not the freshmen.

What I mean to say is that teaching is teaching, no matter the group of students. Responding to the prior or present involvements of the students needs some practical acknowledgement, but does not much affect the basic teaching tasks for you or the basic learning tasks for them. Treat them like adult students; with respect and a firm hand.

6.6 Courses for Non-Architects

I have had some experience in teaching students who are not in the mainstream that this book is basically written for: those in an architecture program in a collegiate-level school of architecture in the United States. I have taught art students in an industrial design program and - for several years - civil engineering students in a selected major that effectively constitutes a minor in architecture.

This presents some special logistical and tactical problems, but is not so much different from teaching generally inexperienced students, whatever the context of their involvements. What it tends to spotlight is your ability to really define your topic in fundamental ways, not just in the familiar jargon and images of the comfortable and conditioned world of the experienced professional.

One of the most challenging - and I modestly claim, inspired - pieces of writing I ever did was a short treatise on the fundamentals of structures. After trying to explain them to several succeeding years of freshman architecture students, I decided to try to present them as if I was talking to my mother-in-law. (About as non-architect a person as I could imagine at the time!). She subsequently read it, and I don't think got much of it, but the standing challenge during the writing made me strip away all my easy language and concentrate on the real ideas I was trying to explain with the text and illustrate with the graphics. No fair talking architecteze or engineereze.

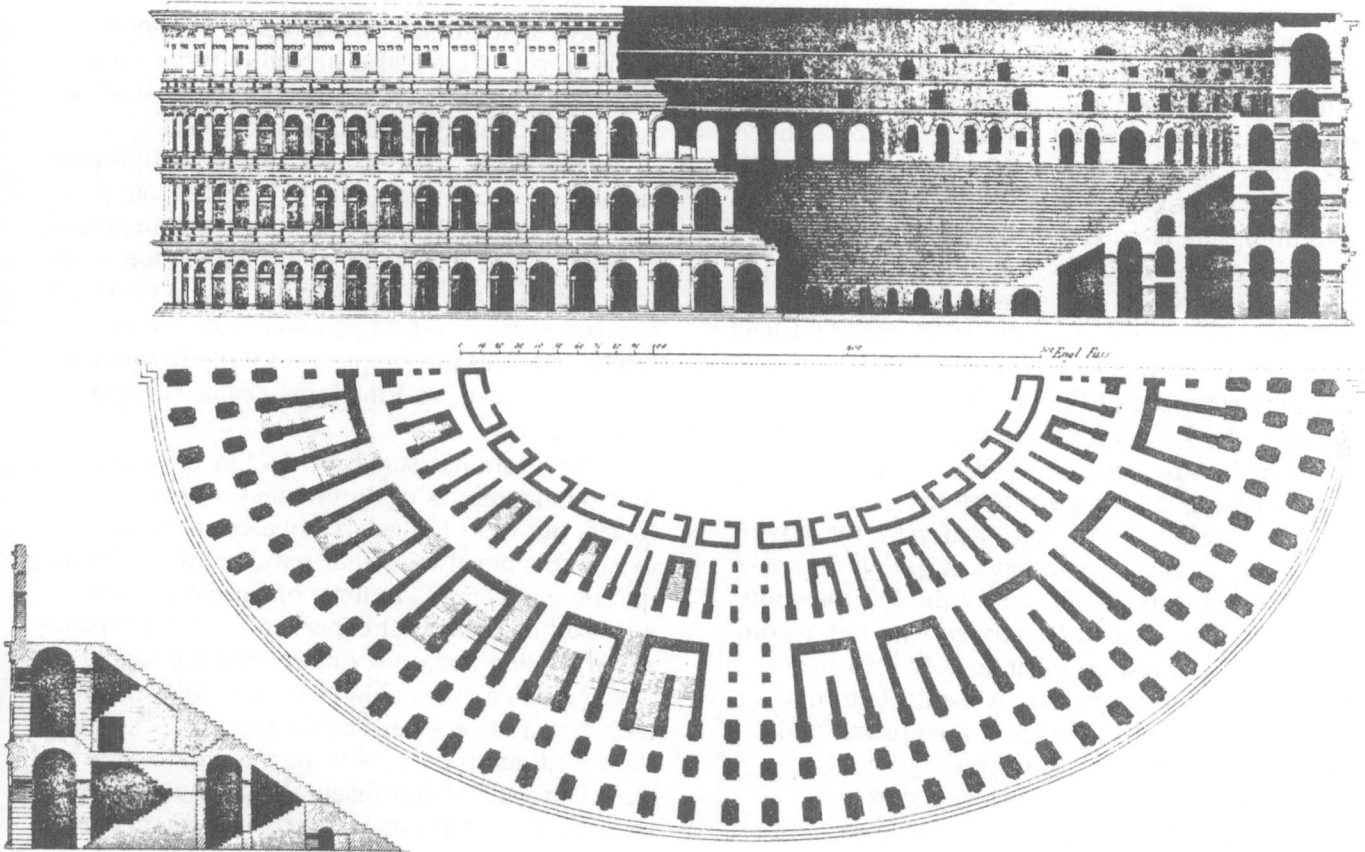

I still like that idea, and sometimes try it even when writing for architecture students or professional architects. Can you explain bending stress in a beam or thermal flow through an exterior wall without resorting to any of the familiar trappings of your trade. It may just come across for the first time to some registered architect.

Here is a place, of course, where the glossary becomes not just a luxury, but an absolute necessity. But keep it painfully short and essential; not as extensive as you can make it. Try coming up with a limited number of terms (say 50) that could be committed reasonably to memory by the students over one hard-study weekend, that will effectively blanket your basic topic. It is a cleansing experience for you and a hard search for the kernel of your real knowledge about the topic. Maybe an embarrassing revelation for you, but good for the educational processes.

6.7   Ad Hoc Courses (Within Studios, Etc.)

Although almost every formal course has some special purposes, the required courses in a professional degree program usually also have a general educational purpose. Thus they have a general topic area that they attempt to cover in some fundamental, comprehensive fashion.

Ad hoc courses are those developed for some more tightly-focused purpose. I have taught a lot of credit-bearing courses with long sequences of lectures, but have also given many one-shot lectures or short series for groups with special needs.

The short treatise on fundamentals of structures that I referred to in the preceding section was an

33

outgrowth of a two-lecture series I gave for several semesters to students in a freshman architecture studio. These students were expected to do some building design projects, but had no other instructional background in the general fields of architectural technology. Their teachers felt they needed some input about basic structures, and conned me into doing the lectures. It was fun, but a very disturbing experience for me, being as smug as I was in my professional grasp of my field.

The ad hoc course is really much more difficult than a full set of semester-long lectures. Given yawning stretches of time to develop the topic, anyone who knows it can spin it out. Try getting it across in a few choice words. Less is more, but it depends a lot on what the less really is.

With painfully short time, and yet a receptive and needy audience, you have to give them something besides talk. (Remember the 5% retention claim?) Have your brilliantly-concise talk recorded on video; make up a handout of your major points; use some book that is available to the students so they can pursue it themselves to the depth they want later; somehow - give them something to work with after you shut up.

Of course, it goes without saying, you have to fully understand the precise, special needs of the ad hoc course. This includes some ability to place yourself in the position of your audience. What do they not know that they need to know and why do they need to know it? You have to get tight with that to make your teaching effort worth the time - yours and theirs. Come to think of it, that is a good question to apply to any teaching effort.

6.8 Exam Blasters

A special ad hoc course is that developed as a review or pumping-up exercise for some exam. The granddaddy of these is the prep course for a professional registration exam. Major businesses are built around this effort for the many such exams, including that for registered architect.

I have given such lecture courses (or seminars) and have written materials intended to support such efforts. I have also helped to write some registration exams. And, incidently, have taken and passed a couple; oral and otherwise.

This represents the essence of directed-purpose: simply, expressly, and only to pass the lousy exam! Learning here is not for any noble purposes; just to beat the exam, to psyche out the exam-writers and graders, and win the day in court. If you buy that, I suggest you start with the exam. Study that, and the people who write it, and the way it is graded, and the legal channels for challenging it.

Every exam has some form. For the three or four day architects exam this means several forms, but most topics are covered in written exams that mostly use four-part, multiple-choice questions. This is the form of the SAT exams, and a lot of high level expertise has been expended on writing and on trying to beat the SATs.

I propose that candidates for the ARE (architects registration exam) could as well spend their time reading up on how to beat multiple-choice exams in general (profusely documented for crashing the SATs) as waste their time studying subject materials for the 8-part ARE. One aspect of the multiple-choice question is that to stand against challenges, it has to have an obvious, unequivocal answer and the wrong answers have to be obviously and unequivocally wrong. In that context, if you can't spot the right answer immediately, you really don't know enough to answer the question intelligently and you have to resort to working on the odds.

Other than that, it is a matter of really bearing down on the kernels of knowledge at the heart of the topics. Less is more, with a real burnoff of the trivial and highly special. Anything available to get that focus may be helpful.

I just happen to have some study aids at the back of my book that are consciously developed with this study concept generally in mind. They are not especially intended for blasting the ARE, but may help some. They are really intended for blasting my course exams and I tell the students so with no reservations. They don't listen, of course (5% retention and all), so my exams remain a major challenge.

7

Basic Course Forms and Work

It is imperative, of course, that teachers get themselves organized and prepared for their contributions to a course. I find, however, that for me it is not any longer a problem; possibly because of my long experience in having to do it. What remains a problem, however, is trying to work out what exactly the students are going to do besides just sit their at attention, soaking up my brilliant lectures (at the usual 5% efficiency). This chapter treats the matter of what the students do.

7.1 Lecture Courses: Schedule, Readings, Tests

The minimum components of a lecture course for me are a schedule, some assigned outside readings, and some test(s). The schedule generally indicates to the students (and to me) what we are going to do and when we are going to do it. It also points out major events: exams, assignment due dates, holidays, etc. I make it as intelligently and thoroughly as possible, but warn the students that modifications are likely because of unanticipated occurrences or some lack of my foresight on what they can or cannot handle.

Accepting the problem of their low retention of lecture-delivered materials, I try to give them an indication of what they have available to use outside of class that covers the lecture topics.

This may include citations from the course text, supplementary handouts, or assigned reading from other books - theoretically available from the library. I avoid the latter as much as possible, because with a large class, somebody frequently steals or tears out the material from the library copy - and that's it for the rest of the class.

It is good that they have something besides the notes from your lecture to use outside of class. Whenever possible, I try to use the text - and select it for the course on that basis - as the real primary source for study. Any text will have some gaps that you will feel obligated to fill with lectures, but the less the students have to depend on the lectures the better, for my purposes. If you really want them to read something else, give them all a personal copy of it somehow in spite of the copyright laws.

Test them often and give their graded tests back as soon as possible for the value of the feedback. Logistically, that means some kind of easy-to-grade tests for a large class, but so be it. The rapid feedback is more important than the intellectual value of the test format.

I am happiest when the nonperforming students all drop before the end of the semester and I don't have to give any flunking grades. I help them all I can to be aware of their bad work at all times to promote this. Of course, I also use the rapid feedback to let them know they need my help, if they will avail themselves of it.

35

I hate final exams for all kinds of reasons, but they do have some useful teaching purposes. Mostly they make the student reflect a bit on what they have learned (or not) during the semester; like getting one more cup of coffee out of the old grounds. In my school finals are required by the university, so I pass the buck for them on up. But I usually make them only a token percent of the course grade.

I love the short single-item quiz. Mostly to stimulate some attendance and actual periodic study. In my construction course, these are usually vocabulary tests over some limited list of words and terms. One chapter's worth or simply a list I give out the period before the quiz.

I don't give a lot of multiple question exams, simply because the scheduled class time is too precious to give up what is available for exams. Still, if the topic scope of the course is broad, you have to let them take serious exams in as small a bite as possible. I usually settle for three exams in a 14 week semester. That means I only lose about 10% of the scheduled class time.

The materials that follow indicate some samples of course schedules, short quizzes, and hour exams. I also include my most recent final exam with a format of multiple choice questions. I have to (theoretically) turn my final grades in within three days after the final exam, so I do a very easy-to-grade final exam. I do, however, take the time to assess the answers and do some statistical correction of the exam. My usual method is to drop any question that at least half of the top 25% of the highest-scoring students miss on the exam. It is to be expected that a lot of the students will miss a tough question, but the top 1/4 of the class shouldn't.

In general academia there is the concept of the course syllabus. Honorable teachers give this out at the beginning of a course to generally explain everything about the course: purpose, meaning, scope, procedures, rules & regulations, grading, required work, lecture topics, schedule, etc. I usually settle for a one page summary of a few basic items - mostly of a more pragmatic nature, like when and where is the class, when and where are my office hours, what is the text, etc. That, together with the course schedule is my syllabus. The following samples are from materials developed for my 3-credit lecture course for second year architecture students.

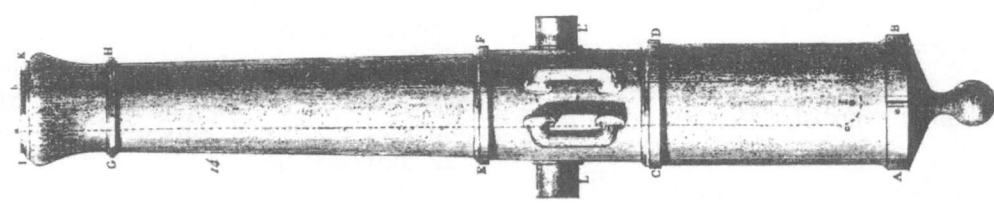

GENERAL INFORMATION FOR THE COURSE

I generally try to keep this to one page, hoping they might actually read it. Anyway, it puts me officially on record with giving them certain basic information. They may not get it because they don't come to class when I hand it out, they may lose it, or they may get it and never read it - the other 5% of the class will get it, keep it, read it, and then forget it. Remind them of important rules every once in a while.

Architecture 211 - Fall 1992

Schedule: 12.00 to 1:20, Tuesday & Thursday

Faculty: James Ambrose, Office - Harris Hall 109
Office Hours - 10:00 - 11:30, Tue. & Thurs.

Text: Building Construction and Design, James Ambrose, Van
Nostrand Reinhold, 1992.

General Description of Course:

This courses deals with issues relating to the construction of
buildings. As a learning experience, the course seeks to
achieve the following:

1. To build awareness of the effects on architectural design of
concern for the proper development of building construction
materials, processes, and details.
2. To develop awareness of the nature of the materials,
products, and systems commonly used for building construction.
3. To develop awareness of current practices in design and
construction of buildings and of the general operations of the
design professions, regulatory agencies, and building industry
in the United States.
4. To develop skills in the use of resources for information
and in the preparation of design communication elements that
relate to the design of building construction.

In the architecture curriculum, this is the first course in the
series of eight courses on building technology, and it has a
secondary purpose to introduce some general concerns for technology
in architecture.

Work done this semester will consist of the following:

Attendance and participation in the class lecture/discussion
sessions.
Quizzes, class-time exams, and the final exam.
Homework assignments.
The semester grade will be determined by evaluation of all the
course work. Approximate grade determination will be as
follows: class participation - 10%, homework - 30%, quizzes -
10%, class-time exams - 30%, final exam - 20%.
Alpha/numeric conversion - A: 90-100, B: 80-89, C: 70-79,
D: 60-69.

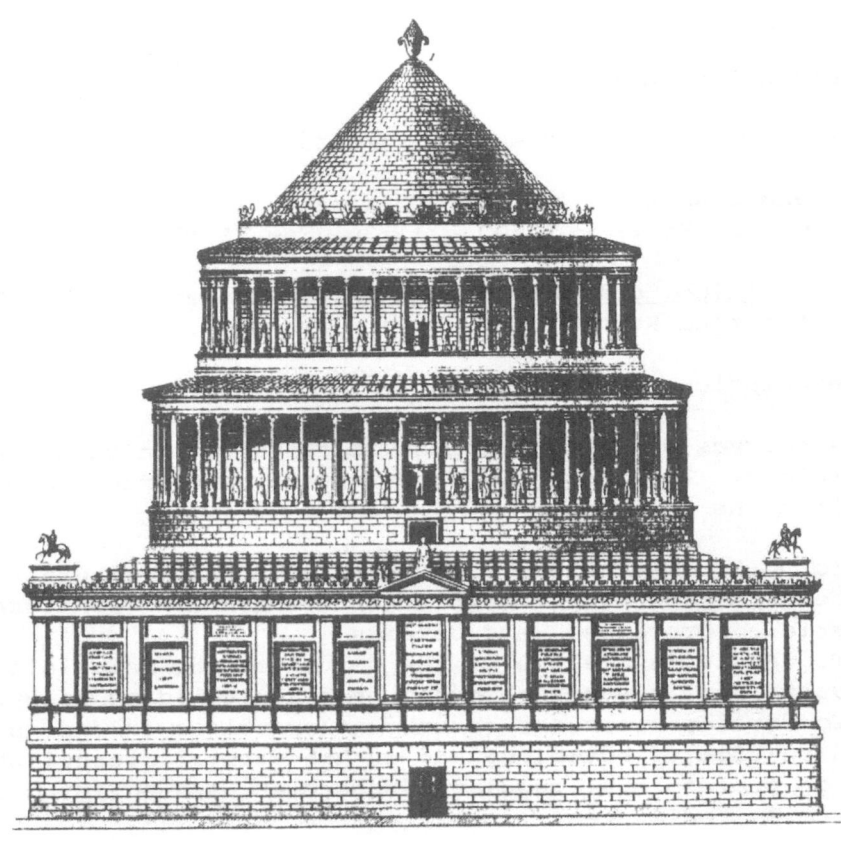

THE COURSE SEMESTER SCHEDULE

This is probably more important to the teacher
than to the students. It helps you to plan your
lectures, reminds you when you need to make up
the assignments, quizzes, and exams, and when
your weekends are going to be ruined by a mountain of grading.

Expect to have to make some changes for
unforseen events. Announce the changes on a
day when hardly anyone attends class - especially
when you extend the due date for an assignment.

The schedule shown on the next page is for a
14-week semester with 80-minute class periods
twice a week (Arch 211). It is an introductory
course for second year architecture students with
no previous technology courses and two previous
semesters of architectural design. The aims of
this course are described in the general course
information sheet shown on the preceding page.

My real preference would be to have two
courses, with my book used for the second
course. The first course would use a text like
Allen's or Watson's to develop the general background of basic construction materials and
processes. The second course would concentrate
on design of construction systems and development of construction details - mostly utilizing the
last chapter of my book to support the kind of
assignments described for 211 or - better yet -
ones as described for the lecture/workshop course
or studio in Section 7.3 of this manual. Dream-
ing on, this would be followed by another studio
or lecture/workshop that consisted of development
of fully integrated building systems (HVAC,
lighting, plumbing, etc.).

```
Arch 211    Fall 92    COURSE SCHEDULE    (As of 9/8/92)


Class-Date        Topic/Event (Text Chapters)    [Quiz]  Assign. (Due)
-------------------------------------------------------------------------

  1    9/1       Introduction
  2    9/3       Construction in Architecture (1-4)
  3    9/8       System 1: Wood Frame   (9,10)                1 (9/29)
  4    9/10          "          (5,6,7,8)           [1]
  5    9/15      Roofs        (7,8,10)
  6    9/17      Doors & Windows (5,7,8)            [2]
  7    9/22      System Development (9,10)          [3]
  8    9/24      Exam 1
  9    9/29      System 2: Concrete & Masonry (9,10)          2 (10/27)
 10    10/1      Concrete     (5,6,7,8)
 11    10/6          "                            [4]
 12    10/8      Masonry    (5,6,7,8)
 13    10/13         "                            [5]
 14    10/15     Foundations   (7)
 15    10/20     System Development   (9,10)       [6]
 16    10/22     Exam 2
 17    10/27     System 3: Steel/Curtain Walls (9,10)         3 (12/1)
 18    10/29     Steel    (5,6,7,8)
 19    11/3      Curtain Walls  (8,9,10)           [7]
 20    11/5          "
 21    11/10     Interior Construction             [8]
 22    11/12         "
 23    11/17     System Development   (9,10)       [9]
 24    11/19     Exam 3
 25    11/24     System Development   (9,10)
Thanksgiving
 26    12/1      Systems Design Concepts (2,3,9)
 27    12/3      Design Documentation   (10)       [10]
 28    12/8      Review

Final Exam:   12/15, 2:00-4:00pm
```

QUIZZES

I try to give these as often as possible. They should relate to some useful module of your presentation and the text. I give them the word list for the quiz the period before. (See the comprehensive word list for the final exam - which is a collection of the word lists for the individual quizzes.)

These are actually mostly to encourage attendance. In my large class they can copy from whomever they choose around them. I don't much care - it is the blind leading the blind. The quiz grade is a small, but real, part of their final grade.

I usually have enough quizzes to be able to drop the one lowest score before averaging the quiz grade at the end of the semester. That typically means they get one free class absence.

Incidentally, I also take attendance on the days they don't have a quiz or exam. That is the main basis for the part of their semester grade called "Class Participation" on the course information sheet. I count a missed quiz as an absence, so it is a double loss.

The quizzes are my main vehicle for promoting the learning of a minimum construction vocabulary. As discussed previously in this manual, I believe strongly in developing the students' vocabulary as a means of gaining a general familiarity with the field of construction.

I also tell the students that the word lists are generally the scope of the questions that will be asked on the exams. The exam questions try to get at something more than rote memorizing of definitions, but that alone is a start toward understanding of the significance of the items on the lists. See the comprehensive word lists for the course, presented here after the example final exam.

Name:_____
first   last

Place the letter corresponding to the correct word or term in front of each definition.

A Species
B Stress graded lumber
C Softwood
D Hardwood
E Veneer
F Oriented strand board

G Waferboard
H Particleboard
I Common nail
J Lag screw
K Split ring connector
L Box beam

____ Compressed wood fiber panels in which wood fibers are randomly placed.

____ Wood from cone-bearing trees.

____ Wood fastener employing a shear (slip) resisting device between the members in a bolted joint.

____ Specific identity of tree from which wood is obtained.

____ Face ply in laminated wood panels.

____ Wood identified for specific structural usage.

____ Compressed wood fiber elements with linear arrangement of wood fibers.

____ Smooth, linear steel element, dynamically inserted to achieve fastening of wood elements.

____ Composite structural element, ordinarily formed with lumber and plywood.

____ Threaded fastener for wood, advanced by torsion in the manner of tightening of a bolt.

IN-CLASS EXAMS

I grudgingly give up two or three class periods per semester to give exams in the class period. These generally cover all the materials developed in the course up to that point or since the last exam. I generally make these a significant part of the course grade, so they are a bit more serious.

In my large class, I usually assemble at least four different versions of each exam, scrambling the layouts of the pages. That way, if they try to copy, it makes it a lot harder.

The multiple choice form is simply easier and faster to grade and lets me return the exams usually at the next class period. The rapid feedback of the exam results is important for them and for me. This also makes a task that can be handed over to an assistant; in my case - typically - my loving spouse.

Rapid feedback and grading efficiency or not, I usually scan the test results for evidence of bad questions. (See discussion for the final exam.) If time permits, I go over the exam questions in class at the time I hand back the exam. I also often write their current course grade status on the exams, so they have a running notice of their situation in the class. The latter often prompts some first-time office counselling.

first   last

Select the response that most correctly completes or answers each of the statements or questions by circling the letter preceding the response.

With a light wood-framed bearing wall, sheathed with plywood, the vertical loads are resisted primarily by the

A   studs   B   studs and the plywood   C   plywood

With a wood-framed shear wall sheathed with plywood, the principal shear-resisting element is the

A   stud system   B   sill plate   C   plywood   D   top plate

Gypsum drywall panelling consists of a sandwich of

A   portland cement plaster and paper   B   plywood and plastic
C   gypsum plaster and plywood   D   gypsum plaster and paper

Cross-grain shrinkage of second floor joists is least likely to be a problem with

A   deep joists   B   platform framing   C   balloon framing

Lumber grades used for light wood framing are usually

A   the lowest feasible   B   the highest available
C   whatever is laying around the lumberyard

Oriented strand board (OSB) is produced for

A   nonstructural applications only   B   wall sheathing only
C   competition with solid wood and plywood

Use of split ring connectors produces joints which

A   are less expensive   B   are less subject to movement
C   require less craft skill

In the United States softwoods are used almost exclusively for light wood framing instead of hardwoods because

A   the wood is stronger   B   the trees are smaller
C   the trees have larger and straighter trunks

43

Select the response that most correctly completes or answers each of
the statements or questions by circling the letter preceding the
response.

In light wood frames, firestops are intended to

A prevent fires   B prevent spread of fires on surfaces
C prevent spread of fires in void spaces   D put out fires

Vents in soffits are intended to

A reduce moisture problems   B prevent heat loss
C provide fresh air to occupants D ventilate wall voids

The connecting device used most often for light wood framing is

A the lag screw   B the common nail   C the bolt   D glue

A box beam is referred to as a composite structural element because of

A its shape   B its use
C its appearance   D the combination of materials

The primary purpose of bridging for joists and rafters is

A achieving of load sharing   B lateral bracing
C reduction of deflection   D alignment of members

The primary reason for having an odd number of plies in plywood is to

A cut costs   B have face plies with the same grain direction
C reduce shrinkage D improve appearance

Use of plank deck results in higher resistance to fire because of

A the species of wood used   B the tighter joints in the deck
C the deck thickness   D the solid sawn wood form

A form of roofing LEAST likely to be effective on a high-slope
(45 degrees or more) roof is

A wood shingle.   B batten-seam metal.
C built-up membrane.   D clay tile.

Name_____
                          first   last

Select the response that most correctly completes or answers each of the statements or questions by circling the letter preceding the response.

The form of window MOST likely to be easily made weather-proof is the

A sliding window.   B casement window.
C fixed window.   D awning window.

The construction element that generally achieves the transition between the rough opening in a wall structure and the precise nature of the window construction is the

A glazing.   B mullion.   C frame   D sash.

The form of glazing intended to reduce heat loss through the glazing itself is

A single glazing.   B laminated glazing.   C double glazing.

A construction element or detail used to secure water resistance at the joint between the roofing edge and the back of a parapet wall is

A a firecut.   B counterflashing.   C a cant.   D a fascia.

Membrane roofing may serve the dual purpose of being the roofing as well as

A a vapor retarder.   B insulation.   C ballast.   D roof deck.

Proper positioning of a vapor retarder in a wall or roof construction is primarily intended to prevent

A excessive heat loss.   B water leaks during precipitation.
C condensation within the construction.   D air leaks.

THE FINAL EXAM

We get a two hour period for our final exams. That permits a size of exam slightly longer than the in-class exam, although I use the same multiple choice format. The questions here are mostly reruns of the in-class exam questions, sometimes rewritten to be a bit trickier.

This exam usually has enough questions for me to do some kind of statistical correction for bad questions. As discussed previously, I usually survey the student success with the individual questions and drop any that seem unfair. My usual method is to drop a question if less than half of the top 25% scorers got it right. I also drop any that I decide have ambiguity between the answer choices after I have given the exam.

I try to have at least 40 questions or so for the two-hour exam. That gives them about three minutes per question, which is about twice the time given for the SAT and the architects registration exam. Am I generous or what?

The word lists given here following the example exam are given out in the last class period. These consist mostly of the lists for the individual quizzes, but may include some material developed in class sessions following the last in-class exam. See the semester schedule.

Name _____
first   last

Circle the letter preceding the correct response.

To accommodate installation of a window, the rough opening in a wall should be

A   Smaller than the frame
B   Larger than the frame
C   The same size as the frame
D   The same size as the sash

Weather seals against air and water are easiest to achieve with a window that is

A   Double hung
B   Horizontally sliding
C   Fixed
D   A casement type

Gypsum drywall panelling consists of a sandwich of paper and

A   Wood fiber board
B   Precast concrete
C   Precast plaster
D   Fiberglass

A principal reason for adding water to a concrete mix is to

A   Reduce unit weight
B   Raise strength
C   Improve workability
D   Speed up hardening

Use of a drip improves the water-related performance of a

A   Vertical mullion
B   Window jamb
C   Horizontal mullion
D   Glazing seal

Site assembly of structural steel frames is mostly achieved by

A   Welding
B   Rivetting
C   Bolting
D   Nailing

Excessive settlement of supports will cause the most damage to a building structure made of

A   Wood
B   Masonry
C   Light-gage steel
D   Fabric

Use of off-site precasting of concrete structures usually results in

A   Lower quality concrete
B   Simpler connections
C   Faster site erection
D   More site formwork

The most effective means for reducing solar heat gain with a window is to

A   Use reflective glazing
B   Use double glazing
C   Shade it on the outside
D   Shade it on the inside

In curtain wall construction, the breaking of a thermal bridge usually results in

A   Collapse of the wall
B   Water leaks
C   Less conductive heat loss
D   Better looking joints

Arch 211   FINAL EXAM

Name _____
                    first   last

Circle the letter preceding the correct response.

In modern structural masonry
construction lintels over wide openings
are usually achieved with

A   Arches
B   Corbels
C   Steel framing
D   Stone blocks

Use of resilient furring for gypsum
drywall on a ceiling or partition is
intended to enhance

A   Fire resistance
B   Sound separation
C   Structural resistance
D   Thermal insulation

Lower cost of concrete structures is
usually achieved by use of

A   More steel and less concrete
B   More concrete and less steel
C   More cement and less water
D   More sand and less gravel

Waterproofing of a curtain wall joint
in which the exact form and dimensions
of the joint are not highly subject to
control will usually be performed with

A   A gasket
B   A membrane
C   A sealant
D   Safing

With the stick method of erection for a
curtain wall, structural attachment of
the wall is made by connecting the
spandrel beams to the

A   Horizontal mullions
B   Vertical mullions
C   Spandrel panels of the wall
D   Window sash units

To reduce glass breakage, the freedom
of movement for glass in curtain wall
systems is usually achieved by

A   Leaving the glass loose in its
     supporting frame
B   Using materials for frames that are
     softer than the glass
C   Inserting soft elements between the
     glass and its frame
D   Using highly flexible materials for
     frames

Preventing the rapid drying of freshly-
cast concrete results in all of the
following EXCEPT

A   Higher concrete strength
B   Shrinkage of the concrete
C   Harder concrete surfaces
D   Less porous concrete

Use of concrete fill on steel floor
decks generally achieves all of the
following as positive effects, EXCEPT

A   Improvement of the fire resistance
     of the construction
B   Improvement of the acoustic barrier
     between interior spaces
C   Reduction of the dead weight of the
     construction
D   Reduction of the bounciness of the
     floor structure

Plywood sheathing on a stud wall is NOT
considered to function to

A   Brace the studs laterally
B   Add to vertical load capacity
C   Develop shear wall resistance
D   Resist direct wind pressure on the
     wall surface

Except for tests performed directly on the structure, the most reliable indicator of strength for finished concrete is the

A Slump test
B 28-day compression test
C Unit density test
C Rorschach test

At the building site, the water content of a concrete mix is commonly tested by

A Weighing the mix
B A compression test
C A slump test
D A density test

The type of foundation element that is located near the ground surface and develops load resistance by vertical bearing pressure is a

A Friction pile
B End-bearing pile
C Footing
D Socketted Caisson

Deep foundation elements generally

A Have low resistance to lateral forces
B Experience major settlements
C Are more economical than bearing footings
D Have low resistance to vertical loads

Building code hourly ratings for fire resistance of construction assemblies are intended to indicate

A Code approval for relative fire resistance
B How long before collapse will occur during a fire
C How long occupants have to get out of the building during a fire
D How long it will take firefighters to put out the fire

One of the most POSITIVE factors for the choice of masonry for building structures is

A Its light weight
B Its low cost
C Its durability
D Its adaptability to structural tasks

One of the most NEGATIVE factors for the choice of masonry for building structures is

A Its fire resistance
B Its compressive strength
C Its natural thermal insulative character
D Its durability

Masonry wall construction with CMUs lends itself to being relatively easily reinforced PRIMARILY due to the

A Hollow form of units
B Nature of concrete
C Form of mortar joints
D Typical multi-wythe construction

The form of wall construction that most effectively uses the thermal inertia potential of masonry for control of interior comfort conditions is one that uses insulation that is

A Applied on the exterior surface
B Applied on the interior surface
C Inserted within hollow masonry units
D Placed between masonry wythes

A construction element or detail used to reduce cracking in masonry walls is a

A Tie
B Cant
C Control joint
D Batten

Circle the letter preceding the correct response.

The rolling process for the production of structural steel shapes typically results in

A Member cross sections with closed forms (tube, cylinder, etc.)
B Steel with considerable hardening and loss of ductility
C Member cross sections with sharp interior corners
D Member cross sections with open shapes

Camber for steel beams is provided to

A Reduce the need for diaphragm action of decks
B Lessen the effect of deflections
C Improve fire resistance
D Prevent rusting of the steel

A construction element essential for prevention of vertical spread of fire with a curtain wall is

A A thermal bridge
B A compression gasket
C Adhesive sealant
D Safing

In an all metal and glass curtain wall system, glazing used to achieve an opaque cover over construction is called

A Single glazing
B Double glazing
C Spandrel glazing
D Laminated glazing

Higher grades of structural steel have

A Greater stiffness
B Greater density (unit weight)
C Greater strength
D Greater fire resistance

Buildings with exposed structures of sitecast concrete have all of the following advantages EXCEPT

A Resistance to fire
B Resistance to weather effects
C Lower total weight
D Resistance to contact with soil

Air-to-air transmission of heat between the exterior and the interior of a building will be least through a window with

A Single strength glass
B Double strength glass
C Single glazing
D Double glazing

With operable windows, the glazing is installed in the

A Rough opening
B Jambs
C Sash
D Sill

With a wood framed shear wall sheathed with plywood, the principal shear-resisting element is the

A Stud system
B Sill plate
C Plywood
D Top plate

Use of split ring connectors produces joints which

A Are less expensive
B Are less subject to structural movement
C Require less craft skill
D Are not as strong as ordinary bolted joints

Word List - Arch 211, Final Exam

WOOD

Species   Waferboard
Stress graded lumber   Particleboard
Softwood   Common nail
Hardwood   Lag screw
Veneer   Split ring connector
Oriented strand board   Box beam
Plywood

LIGHT WOOD FRAME

Balloon frame   Bridging
Platform frame   Let-in bracing
Firestop   Eave
Joist   Fascia
Rafter   Soffit
Sheathing   Gypsum drywall

ROOFS

Vapor retarder   Liquid-applied roof membrane
Condensation   Single-ply roof membrane
Batten seam   Built-up roof membrane
Standing seam   Ballast
Cant   Deck
Counterflashing   Tile
Fascia   Shingle
Parapet   Low-slope roof

DOORS AND WINDOWS

Sill   Glazing
Head   Double glazing
Jamb   Window types:
Mullion   Double-hung
Sash   Single-hung
Frame   Sliding
Rough opening   Casement
Thermal behavior   Awning
                                         Fixed

Word List - Arch 211, Final Exam

CONCRETE

Admixture
Aggregate
Air-entraining
Curing
Design compressive strength
Portland cement
Precast construction

Prestressed concrete
Reinforced concrete
Sitecast construction
Slump test
Water-cement ratio
28-day compressive strength
Shrinkage

MASONRY

Wythe
Veneer
Reinforced masonry
Mortar
Masonry unit
Grout
Tie

Furring strip
Face brick
CMU
Cavity wall
Bearing wall
Lintel

FOUNDATIONS

Cohesive soil
Cohesionless soil
Compaction
Differential settlement
Shallow-bearing foundation
Deep foundation

Footing
Friction pile
End-bearing pile
Belled caisson
Socketted caisson

STEEL

Grade (of steel)
Angle
Arc welding
Channel
Cold working
Composite construction
Drawing
Formed decking

Camber
High-strength bolt
Hot-rolling
Moment connection
Open web joist
Shear connection
Wide flange section
Buckling

Word List — Arch 211, Final Exam

CURTAIN WALLS

Cladding
Double glazing
Drip
Extrusion
Gasket
Mullion

Safing
Sealant
Spandrel
Stick system
Thermal bridge
Unit system

INTERIORS

Hourly fire ratings
Flame spread
Acoustic separation
Resilient furring
Nonstructural wall

Demountable partitions
Open planning
Suspended ceiling
Integrated ceiling
Elevated floor

SYSTEMS DESIGN

Hierarchy
Subsystem
Suboptimization
Primary elements
Secondary elements

Systems integration
Mixed systems
Predesigned systems
Structural interference
Modifiable systems

DESIGN DOCUMENTS

Construction drawings
Specifications
Masterformat system
Design contract
Construction contract

Design liability
Plan
Elevation
Section
Notation

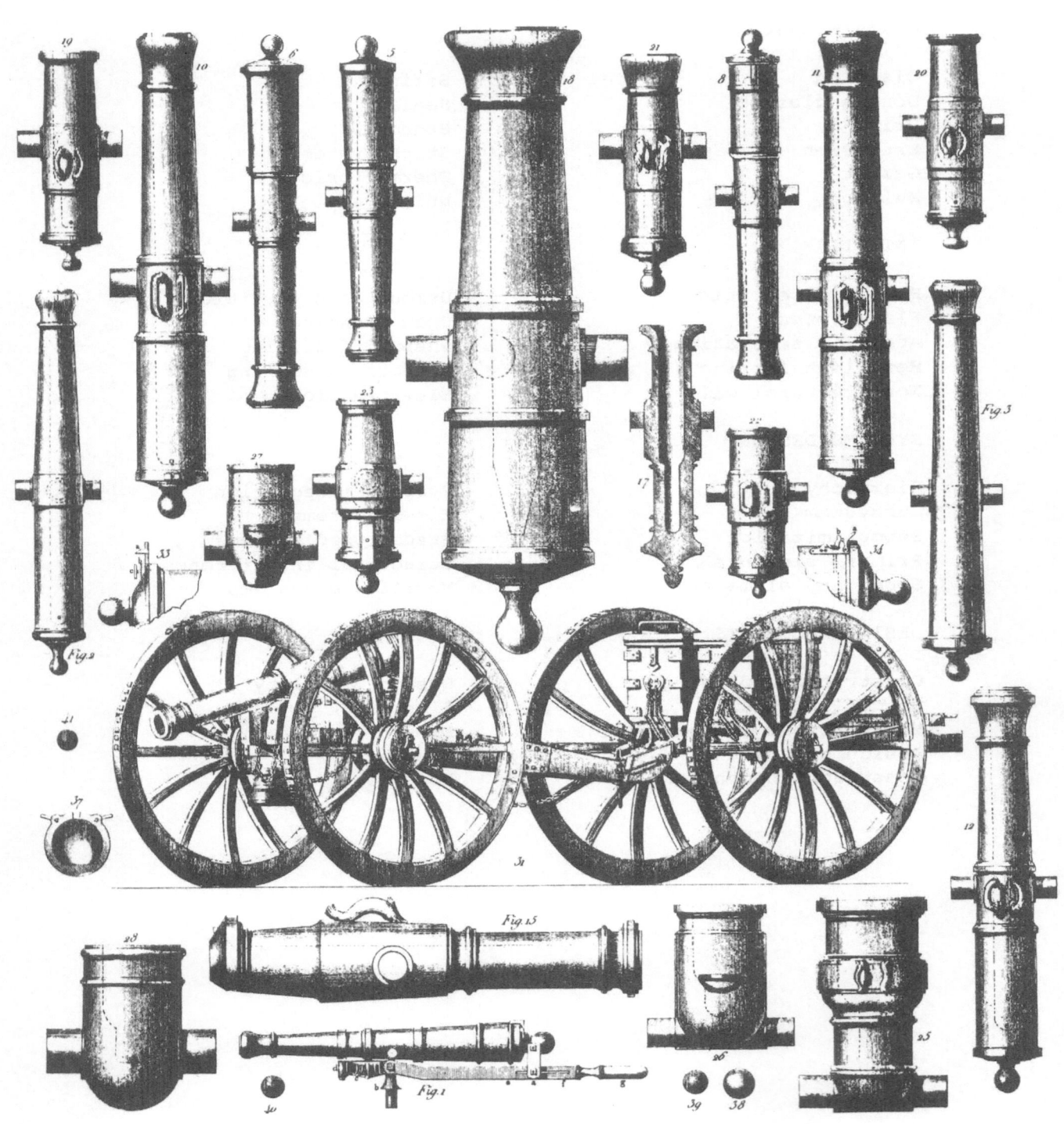

7.2 Lecture Course Assignments

I hate to have to base a course grade entirely on class attendance and test scores. It favors and encourages the diligent, academically-achieving students and raises the GPA average for the school, but does not seem to me to be in the mainstream of architectural education.

Work given in the form of assignments completed outside the lecture classroom have some potential for letting the students work at their own pace, when they want to, and where and how they want to. It also puts them out on their own to do the work and find what they need to do it with. Assuming someone else doesn't do it all for them, this is a potentially much greater challenge and a richer learning experience. I don't think that much of what is important to an architectural designer can be picked up from studying textbooks and taking tests on them.

The kind of assignments I would really like to give in a construction course have more place in a studio than in a lecture course. The typical course scheduling, student/teacher ratio, and general commitment of the students to the course all make it really difficult, if not totally unfeasible, to do this in a lecture course.

Still, after many bruises and scars, I insist on trying. And every semester a handful of students come back to say that they have to admit that the annoying assignments were really the most significant learning experiences in the course. As long as I get a little feedback like that, I will go on submitting myself to the moaning, weeping, cheating, late submissions, lame excuses, and the mountain of grading that this kind of assignment work produces.

I consider the assignments to be the only real opportunity to make the students see even a little bit that the topic has something to do with design work. In fact, the type of assignments shown here have several purposes, having to do with the particular situation in my course and school. Some of these considerations are as follows:

There are no drafting courses, so most of the students don't really know how to make cut section details or, much, how to do orthographic projection in general. I really have to explain what a cut section is. This may be the only real instruction - or experience - they get.

My course is the only one in the curriculum giving basic instruction in construction materials and processes and the development of construction details for buildings.

I prefer to grade tests on a numeric basis - adjusting to a letter grade scale only seriously at the end of the course. However, I prefer to grade assignments on a letter grade basis, as it makes it clearer what I view as the quality of the work in relation to the course letter grade. It also usually raises the student's numeric grade average, as even a D grade is by my alpha/numeric conversion a 65. If they do scarcely anything at all for the assignment, they get at least a D. If they don't do the assignment they get a zero - which establishes my attitude about doing the required course work.

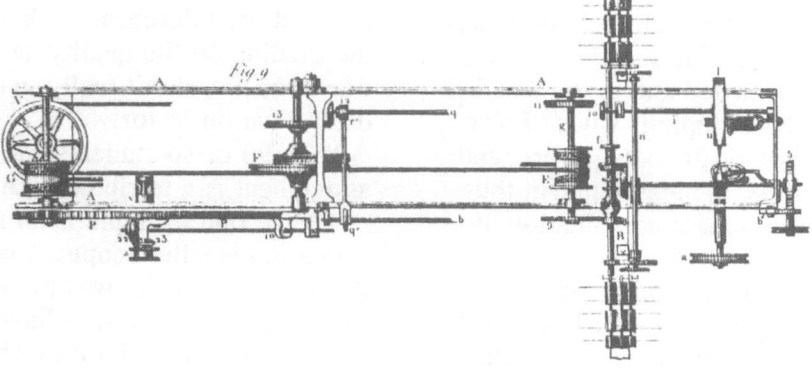

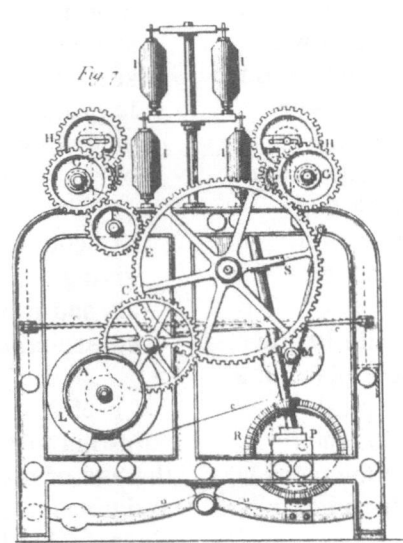

LECTURE COURSE ASSIGNMENT

The first example is an assignment given to students at the beginning of the class involvement in wood construction. It is due shortly after we complete the lectures on wood and go on to other topics. Although the basic topic is wood, I also bring in general discussions of roofs, doors, and windows during this time. The assignment thus relates somewhat to the general combination of the topics.

This is the first assignment, and for many students - the first time they will ever have tried to draft up some construction details. Without using too much class time, I have to discuss drafting, orthographic projection, standard symbols and notation, and all the library resources at their disposal for reference. I also try to comment in the grading on the quality and correctness of their drawings, but don't really make it a major grade determination factor.

With 90 or so students and only little me, this assignment is a terrible chore to grade.

The second example is an assignment with a somewhat smaller scope. I would more likely use this in a course that was the first in a two-course sequence. In my case, I have only one semester, so I zap right into the idea of systems.

Arch 211   F 92   ASSIGNMENT ONE

This assignment consists of the development of the typical details of the construction for a wood framed residential building. The model for the work is the presentation of the case study for Building 1 in the text.

You must select a real building as the basis for this assignment, and your choice may not be the same as that of any other student in the class. You may choose a local building and present photos to generally describe the building. You may also pick a building from a book or magazine article and use the photos and general architectural plans as part of your presentations. Your construction details, however, should be your own original drawings.

The building should have a basic light wood frame or timber frame structure. Otherwise, some difference should be evident in the details by comparison with those in the course text. Use the text for a reference, but not for straight copying.

For the building:

1. Describe the building as to location, use, general form, exterior appearance, etc. Do this with illustrations consisting of sketches and/or photos and a minimum of written comments.

2. Draw cut section details of the exterior construction, illustrating all of the following situations, as applicable.

   Top, bottom, ends, corners, and intersections of the basic exterior construction.

   Intersections of the walls with the roof and floor construction.

   Typical details for a window - head, sill, and jamb.

3. List references you use in developing the details.

It is to be expected that you must be creative in developing these details, but they should be realistic, should represent typical construction, and look like they relate to the building you described.

Present your work on one side of 8.5 X 11 paper, bound in a brochure or notebook. Do not put your pages in plastic sleeves, unless you also provide a copy for my grading notes. Place your work in a 10 X 13 envelope with your name, the Course No., and the Assignment No. on the outside. Submit your original work, but make a copy for your own records before submitting the assignment. Assignment is due in class on October 13.

Arch 211   F 90   ASSIGNMENT ONE

This assignment consists of an analysis of a window. Find a window in
a real building that is of some interest to you and do the following:

    Illustrate its general appearance from both the exterior and
    interior. Use either photographs or line drawings.

    Draw conventional section details of the sill, jamb, and head.
    Show the complete window and wall constructions.

    Describe any special features (hardware, decoration, type of
    glazing, etc.) not clearly shown by your photos and/or drawings.

It is to be expected that you can not really know the details of the
construction, so you must make them up. Use something real as a
reference and list the actual reference sources.

(Presentation requirements as for the preceding assignment.)

7.3 "Design" Assignments

There is really no parallel anywhere in academia for the architectural design studio. I don't speak just of the concept of an individual studio course and its logistics or methodology - although that alone is quite unique. Most students in collegiate programs that may be headed for some career in "design" in art, engineering, or other fields hardly ever have a course of the comprehensive nature of an architectural design studio. So it is already unique in that aspect.

Adding to that unique nature as an educational unit or component is the prominence given to such courses in the architecture school. Despite any idealistic claims by schools, deans, or faculty, the design studios dominate all architecture programs. By mandate (to obtain accreditation by the NAAB) there needs to be a certain critical mass (total credits, total number of courses) of studios in the architecture curriculum and the student teacher ratio has to be below half of what it averages in most universities.

While having just one course like an architecture studio is highly unusual in any other university programs, having a long sequence of them is not conceivable. Yet, in architecture schools, for the accredited undergraduate degree (bachelor of architecture) there are usually at least six or more sequential studio courses. (In my school there are ten - one every semester of the five-year, B Arch program.)

To bring the total amount of studio courses and the student/teacher ratio up to NAAB standards, the studio budget portion of the architecture school's total budget takes up the vast majority of the pie. The vast majority of architecture faculty teach studio courses and the vast majority of space in the school is occupied by studios. Whatever else the school is up to (teaching the architecture lecture courses, service courses to the university, extension work, research?), it seldom adds up to outweigh the expenditures for manning the studios.

This is a context that the development of other course offerings in the architecture program must relate to. For my discussion here, the issue is what kind of work can be done by you and the students in a lecture course as compared to a studio course.

The simple mechanics of the situations must be acknowledged: total scheduled class time, student/teacher ratio, type of classroom space, total credit hours of the class.

The basic nature of the lecture course with a large enrollment (50+) is one of mass-production efficiency. The basic nature of the studio with a small enrollment and long class periods (15 or so students/teacher, two to three hours of class per credit) is an emphasis on close, one-on-one, student-teacher contact and intense intra-class student interaction.

The basic form of assignment work that can be undertaken by the students, and handled for development and grading by the teacher, is miles apart for the two course situations. Logistics alone are not what characterizes studios in comparison with lecture courses. But the simple mathematics of the logistics must be acknowledged. Added to that, the studios are supposed to deal with different work: of a comprehensive, heuristic, creative, "design" nature. Emulating to some extent the situation in a professional design situation.

I am not against the studios; I think they are essential to architectural education and truly ought to be dominant in the architecture curriculum. I have taught in them; from the beginning to the graduate level. But I think there is a lot that can't feasibly be done in studios, so the curriculum also needs other, limited-topic, didactic, lecture-form courses. The problem is to develop the whole curriculum so that the studios and the "other" courses don't contend in terms of student's motivation and allegiance, teacher respectability, budget, political strength in the school, etc. They need each other and they ought to show it.

So - what I really mean to get to here is what can be done for construction education in a studio context, accepting the situation as I have described it. My view is simple: make it have a design nature and some broader involvement. One way to do that is simply to do some kind of building planning and design exercise that is carried further into the definitive design development stage; maybe even in a token way into final

59

(working drawings and specs) stages. Or, if the Bauhaus can be resurrected, into actually building something; preferably the real thing, but maybe at least a model.

I can't really help you here if you haven't ever taken - or better yet, taught - a studio course. If you have taught studios, I think you can easily visualize in theory the possibility of carrying simple design projects into this level of development. Not for some fantastically complicated, urban complex, but for a single, not too big or complicated building.

With six or more sequential studio courses in an architecture curriculum, a possibility would be to make then ascend in sequence by treating, steadily ever more fully, the stages of the architectural design process. Thus, the first studio would deal only with the earliest, most information-deprived, free expressions of the designers imagination. Maybe not even architecturally-appearing problems at all, but basic design concepts of form, scale, space, perception, simulation, symbolism, structure, etc. Learn these things fundamentally, without having to associate them with housing density, building codes, material properties, or construction processes.

But the last studio in the curriculum should require carrying the "design" work into some token development of construction drawings and specifications. Spanning the whole spectrum from concept to reality. Getting to that point of capability would require a lot of inputs along the way (lecture courses, sequential buildup of involvement and complexity in the studios, case studies of actual building designs). But - hey - we have five years of architecture school to do it, don't we?

Oh well!

Give me just one construction course (not the first; maybe the third or so) that is studio-like in nature. With the classroom space, scheduled time, credit hours, and student/teacher ratio to be able to do studio-like work. And then we can do something like design work for the teaching of construction in the way that architects will really encounter it in professional practice.

If not, be realistic about what can be accomplished in lecture courses.

7.4   Short Courses

Somewhere short of the studio type of course, and even short of the usual full semester lecture course, is the possibility for some kind of short lecture series on construction. These may have various particular purposes, including the following:

STUDIO SUPPORT. A short series of lectures for a group of students in a studio may be used to input some major topic development tailored to the specific involvements of the studio work. This may be a refresher or a supplement for presentations developed in other courses taken by the students.

My book could be used for this by simply selecting materials related to the specific limitations of the studio assignment. A highrise building, for example; for which the lectures would focus on curtain walls, elevators, and other issues, and review the case studies of the multistory buildings in Chapter Ten.

PREPARATION FOR REGISTRATION. Cramming for the architects registration exam (ARE) is often facilitated by lecture or seminar courses. These are more effective if some study materials are available; to be used during the course and for extended study after the course.

My book is reasonably comprehensive for this purpose - for the construction portion of the ARE. The study aids at the back of the book can be used for classroom and self-study support.

PROFESSIONAL UPDATES. A course offered for the updating of working professionals on the current issues in construction may be built around some initial comprehensive view of what construction for buildings is fundamentally all about - at least from an architect's view.

My book is well oriented and reasonably comprehensive for this purpose. The lectures, of course, would take off from the book to point out what is new and emerging in the technology, research, new building code regulations, latest law suits, etc.

Most effective would be some set of notes for the lecture series that works in conjunction with the book and summarizes the update materials; functioning effectively as an update of the book. If anyone out there undertakes such an effort, I would be very happy to see it.

7.5 Independent (Guided) Studies

Many people undertake to study a topic on their own; with or without any kind of help from other persons. We have all picked up books, videos, or other aids to do this to some extent.

My book lends itself to some degree for use in a self-study effort. The Study Aids at the back of the book are partly developed with this in mind, serving somewhat as a study guide. They can't replace a teacher or mentor, but may help the uninformed to focus on what to concentrate on and what to try to get out of the book materials.

Other than some guidance about what is supposed to be learned, what self-studiers need most is somebody to ask questions of and possibly somebody to prompt them to keep at it. This is basically the role of a teacher, and may occur with a student who enrolls in some kind of independent study course. Over the years, I have dealt with several students in this sort of effort.

Within a semester schedule, what a self-study student needs is mostly what students in regular courses need: some hard schedule, some periodic nudging to keep up the study, some periodic examination for progress and accomplishment, and some opportunity to ask questions. What I mean is, the self-study course should be as organized as, and kept to a schedule as, a regular semester-long course. If you have to handle this, I suggest making a "contract" with the student before the work starts so that the exact purpose, expectation for accomplishment, schedule for study, and periodic contacts are very specifically spelled out and agreed to.

Since self-study in a school is often undertaken because regular course offerings do not provide the desired learning opportunity, there are likely to be some specialized purposes for the undertaking. My book may be used for a takeoff point and general backup for specialized study, but some specific list of other resources should also probably be established to more fully support the special study work. Itemizing those resources should be part of the initial "contract", as the feasibility of the undertaking may depend on their access.

8

General Sources for Study of Construction

Other than your brilliant lectures, there are various sources from which some information about construction can be obtained for learning by the students. This chapter has some comments on the use of the most ordinary of these, in the context of a typical lecture course situation.

8.1 Books

I love books, I own a lot of them, I write some, and I use them personally to learn from. However, they have various limitations, such as:

You can't very easily ask them questions. They may ask themselves some (as I do in the Study Aids section in my book), but it is not quite the same as a face-to-face question opportunity.

They are not very fresh with information. Most of them take several years to write and a year or so to get to market after they are written. Then, they may age well, like fine wine, but probably just slowly rot away with regard to timely information. Watch the evening news if you want timely information; don't look for it in any book.

They are expensive and should be invested in like you would any other long term possession; or maybe a short term, urgently needed one.

There are at any time probably thousands of books in print about some aspect of building construction. It is difficult to find out about all of them and is a real test of your library-use skills. You have to use whatever sources you can to find out about them; especially about new ones on the market or forthcoming ones.

If any professional magazine or association puts out a list of recommended sources, it is about as good as you can expect to find. Advertising hype may cloud the ability to fairly evaluate a particular book. So may the personal viewpoint, prejudices, or jealousies of a single individual reviewer or compiler of bibliographies.

There are a handful of books about building construction in general. I have previously mentioned my two favorites: **Fundamentals of Building Construction**, by Ed Allen and **Construction Materials and Processes**, by Don Watson. Another with a storehouse of information about light construction is **Construction Principles, Materials, and Methods**, by Olin, Schmidt, and Lewis.

If you want some depth in the area of general building construction I suggest getting my book first - then get the other three I have mentioned. They will really compliment each other in many ways and provide a terrific scope of subject coverage. Dated, but comprehensive. Cough up the $200 or so, or look for second hand copies. Whichever one you use as a text, the others will have various better coverage of selected topics.

Beyond that, the plunge is deep, and depends on your special interests. A particular area of concern to me is that of details of building construction. Resources for this are difficult to provide for students. I recommend **Architectural Graphic Standards**, despite its spotty coverage, lack of timeliness, and clumsy organization (the 16-part CSI system). It simply has such a monumental collection of information. With its large pages, its graphics reduced from larger originals, and its virtual bulk, there is a total of graphic information equal to that in about five typical books. Despite its enormous cost, if you divide it by five for comparison with other books, it is a really good investment. But don't treat it with undue respect (in spite of the imprimatur of the AIA); it's just another book.

Despite its even more dated nature, the Student Edition of Graphic Standards (based on the previous, 1980 7th edition) is probably OK for students' needs and a bargain at its price. About 60% of the whole book at about 1/3 the price.

If you want an even more intensive resource, specifically for construction details, I suggest the recently published abridgement of the 8th edition of Graphic Standards, titled **Construction Details from Architectural Graphic Standards**. This has all the details (about half the total pages) from the book and sells for about half the price. A bargain if all you want are details.

My construction book presents a lot of details in the example buildings in Chapter Ten. While reasonably sufficient to explain the buildings, however, they do not remotely constitute a comprehensive resource of all the possibilities, even for the limited set of example buildings. I like to have the students pursue the other possibilities, and make it part of the work on the homework assignments I give in my course. Providing them with, or guiding them to, resources for that information is a major problem.

8.2 Industry Catalogs & Ads

It is assumed that any architecture school library has a set of **Sweets Catalog Files** (the green ones). Maybe not the latest edition, but it is not very important; the scope of materials is what counts. Learning to find things in it is a major homework assignment objective for my students.

Actual copies of individual brochures for class handout may be obtained from some sources, but if they really want to give you that many copies, it is probably material you don't really want to use. Anyway, I think that forcing the students to go out and find this kind of information on their own is an important learning experience. It is a confrontation with the industry, the advertising business, the generic language of the CSI Masterformat System, etc. Traumatic, but a necessary dose of reality sometime.

A warning here - if you send 50+ students to find one page in the library's one copy of Sweets for vital information, one of them will surely tear it out and keep it.

I personally maintain a file of this kind of stuff that I build up by sending in the reply cards from the card decks or the tear-out cards from my magazines. Once in awhile I xerox a page or two from them for my class. But mostly, I use it for my own personal information, since I don't qualify for (or want to spend the money for) my own copy of Sweets.

In my working days (not that long ago), it was next to impossible to get any recommended construction details from the industry. Now you have to beat them away with a club. I am not sure what is the worse situation: a vacuum or a glut. I suggest, however, that if you want to develop your own details for something, that you at least start with whatever the appropriate industry recommends. They may inundate you with

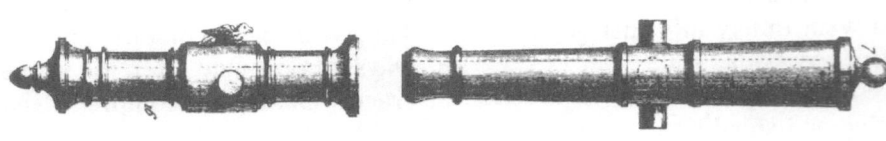

free stuff or offer to sell you a whole library. Ask the roofers how to install roofing; don't try to wing it.

In any event, let the students know that the development of construction details is an art; for the practice of which, people are required to become registered with the state. It is not fully subject to being canned and filed once and for all.

8.3   Visual Aids

Use of visual aids depends on your personal teaching technique and some logistics regarding the classroom, available projection equipment, etc. (See my discussion in Section 3.4 of this manual.) It also depends on what else you have to fill up the class time with. I mostly use visual aids to fill some of the less critical class time.

There are a lot of movies, videos, film strips (now old fashioned), and slide sets available from the industry and various commercial sources. You can easily fill up a whole semester's worth of class time with them, if you really don't like to lecture.

A kind of presentation I find quite useful is one that shows in a short time the sequence of construction for some building, preferably from the virgin site to the occupied building. With a lot of shots of the raw construction along the way. These are great for illustrating the actual construction process and the form of the various subsystems that are out of view in the completed building. Also the confusing mess of a typical construction site.

Actually, I have sometimes given students an assignment of doing such a visual study with photographs over the time span of a semester for some selected building under construction. It is

tough to manage this, however, when they don't really know what to look for, or when the work doesn't really progress much in the limited time of one semester. Still, for students with no previous exposure to actual construction, it is a rich experience.

One possible enrichment for a course is to show slides from your own work, or simply from projects for which you have some personal knowledge. These may be developed as extensions from, or elaborations on, the presentations in the text or the classroom lectures.

Architects and architecture students tend to be quite visually-oriented, so this is a way to entertain them, if the material is at all well presented. However, the real learning purpose and effectiveness must be carefully considered for the value of the time it takes from other classroom involvements and the use of the limited class scheduled time.

8.4   Field Trips

There is really scarcely any substitute for looking at real buildings - completed or under construction. Taking a group of students to building sites and talking about what they are seeing while there is a rich learning opportunity. Doing this with 50+ students in a lecture course is logistically impossible.

If you have a studio, with the smaller group of students as well as a long scheduled class period, it may be conceivable. If your lecture-course students are taking a studio field trip, you may be able to tag along and make some use out of it, during or after the trip.

One variation on this is the self-conducted field trip. I have sometimes made up a map and a

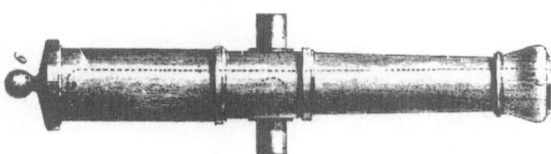
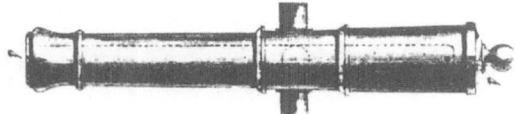

walking tour (maybe of the campus) with some notes about what to look at along the way. Then I somehow get the students to take the tour on their own and report back some way. Or I simply have a discussion with them about the tour, letting them ask questions if they have any.

Or, I simply tell them about various buildings I know about around the campus that have something to see relating to what we are studying. If they are curious enough about them, they go to see them, and sometimes come back with questions.

This sort of thing is of some value for the simple therapeutic effects; breaking down the walls of the classroom and the dry restrictions of the text as a learning source. Don't do it, however, unless you are prepared to answer some questions and use some class time to capitalize on the experiences. And really do take the tour yourself, to anticipate some questions.

Besides looking at buildings, a trip to a brickyard, precast concrete casting yard, steel assembly plant, or other such place can be quite valuable. If you are concentrating on some in-depth look at a selected material or form of construction, this can really intensify the student involvement with the topic.

I have found it to be increasingly difficult to do field trips because of the liability problems. It is next to impossible to get onto construction sites, especially with groups of people. Likewise for factories, unless they have some canned tours that probably don't fit your interests well. A substitute may be a good, short, movie or video from the industry.

Epilogue

ABOUT CARING AND SHARING

If you really read through this manual, you must have some reasonable interest and concern for the teaching of building construction. If so, and you actually use my book for some teaching effort, I would be delighted to hear from you. You can reach me through my school, the University of Southern California in Los Angeles, or my publisher, Van Nostrand Reinhold in New York.

Anyone teaching building construction at an architecture school in the United States should be on the list for Ed Allen's newsletter which is distributed by his publisher, John Wiley & Sons in New York. Ed is really serious about teaching, about construction, and about sharing information and experiences with other teachers.

I also suggest that you try to attend the Teacher's Workshops or the Annual Technology Conference sponsored by the ACSA. This is an unparalleled opportunity for meeting other teachers.

Below are some addresses for capitalizing on these opportunities.

James Ambrose, Professor
School of Architecture
University of Southern California
Los Angeles, CA 90089-0291

or
James Ambrose, Author
c/o Van Nostrand Reinhold
115 Fifth Avenue
New York, NY 10003

Edward Allen, Author
Professional, Reference & Trade Group
John Wiley & Sons
605 Third Avenue
New York, NY 10058-0012

Association of Collegiate Schools of Architecture
1735 New York Avenue NW
Washington, DC 20006

Index